The Complete Knee Pain Relief Cookbook

Simple Recipes for Natural Knee Healing at Home

By: Martha Stanford

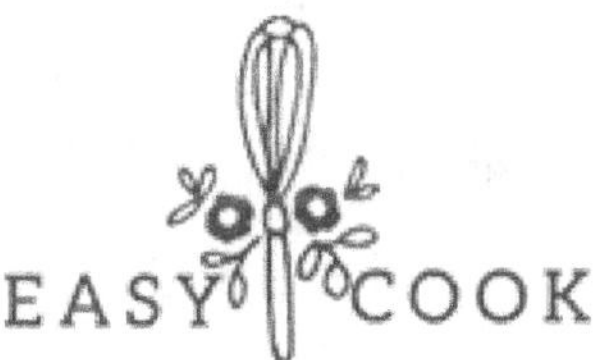

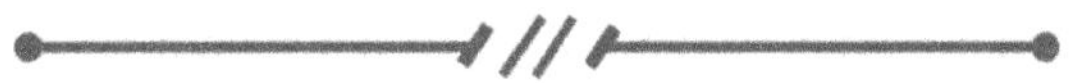

Important Notice

Dear Valued Reader,

This book is the result of my hard work and dedication. I kindly ask that you respect my intellectual property rights by not reproducing, distributing, or transmitting any part of this publication in any form or by any means without my prior written consent. This includes photocopying, recording, or using electronic or mechanical methods. However, brief quotations used in critical reviews and certain other noncommercial uses are permitted by copyright law.

I have put a great deal of effort into ensuring that the information provided in this book is both accurate and useful. However, I cannot guarantee specific results or outcomes from applying this information, as individual circumstances may vary. It is important to remember that you have the power to make your own choices and determine the path that is right for you. While I hope that the content of this book will inspire and guide you, ultimately, the way you choose to use this information is up to you.

By reading this book, you acknowledge that I shall not be held responsible for any consequences resulting from the use or misuse of the information presented.

Thank you for your understanding and for respecting the time and effort I have put into creating this work.

Table of Contents

Introduction

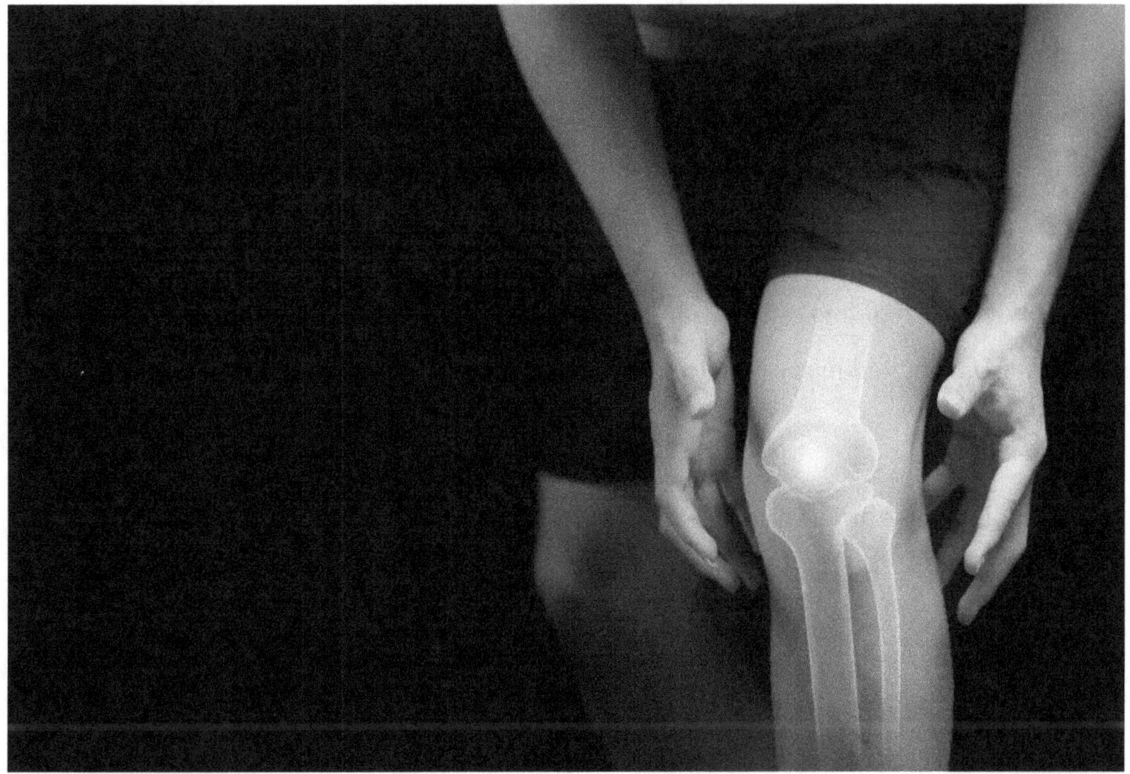

Welcome to your guide for natural knee pain relief. This book is packed with easy-to-make remedies that can help ease your aches without relying on store-bought pills or creams.

Have you ever wondered if there's a gentler way to treat knee pain? Many of us reach for over-the-counter medicines when our knees hurt. But these quick fixes often come with unwanted side effects, especially if used too often.

That's where this book comes in. Here, you'll find a collection of homemade recipes for balms, salves, creams, and rubs. These natural remedies are designed to soothe your knees using ingredients you might already have in your kitchen or can easily find at a local store.

Why choose these homemade options? For starters, they work fast and use natural ingredients. They can help reduce stiffness, improve blood flow, and ease swollen joints. Plus, you can adjust the recipes to suit your needs or preferences.

The remedies in this book aren't just for knee pain. Many can help with other aches and pains too. Whether you're dealing with arthritis, recovering from a tough workout, or just feeling the effects of a long day, you'll find something here that can help.

Making your own pain relief products puts you in control. You'll know exactly what's going into each recipe, avoiding unnecessary chemicals or additives. It's a more natural approach to managing pain, and many people find it more effective than store-bought options.

So, let's get started on your journey to healthier, happier knees. With these recipes, you'll have a toolkit of natural remedies at your fingertips, ready to help whenever aches and pains strike. Happy mixing!

XXXXXXXXXXXXXXXXXXXXXXXXX

1. DIY Knee Pain Salve

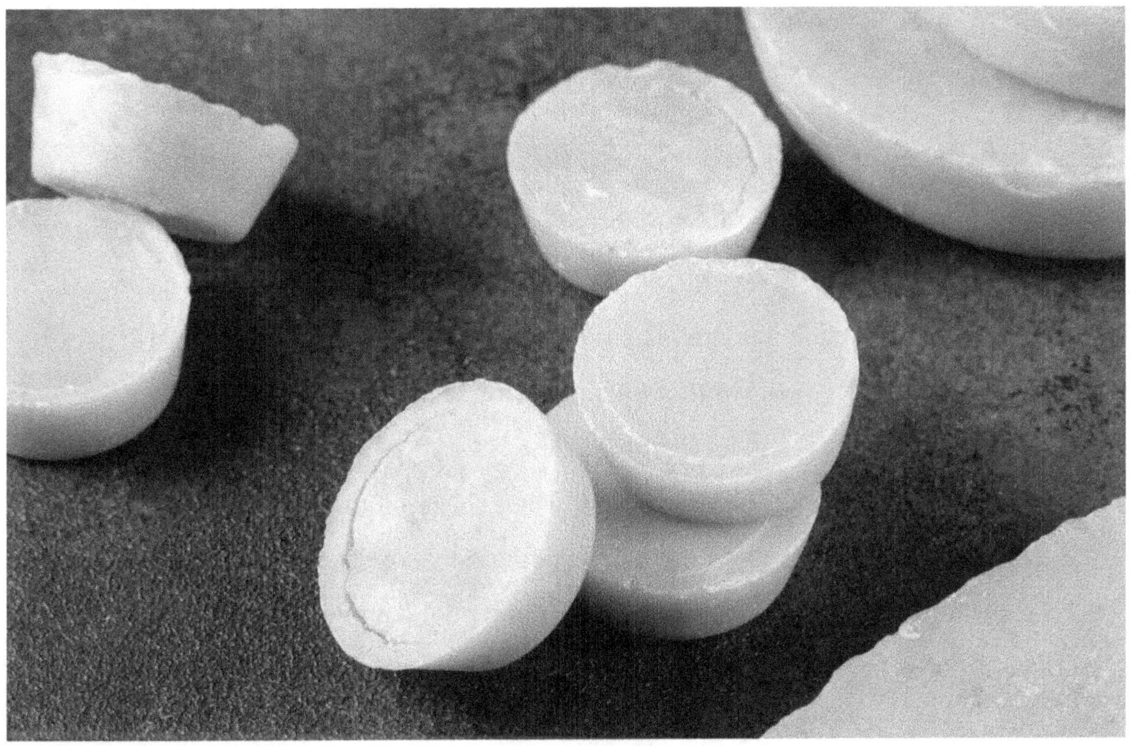

This homemade remedy is great for soothing sore knees after outdoor activities. It's a mix of natural ingredients that work together to ease pain. People love it because it's easy to make and really helps. You'll find it useful after long walks or working in the garden.

Preparation Time: 15 minutes + 24 hours setting time

Serving size: About 4 ounces

Ingredients:

- 4 oz St. John's wort oil
- 2 tsp cayenne powder
- 5 oz beeswax

XXXXXXXXXXXXXXXXXXXXXXXXX

Instructions:

A. Put oil and cayenne in a double boiler. Warm it up gently.
B. Let it cool down, then warm it up again. Don't let it bubble.
C. Take it off the heat and let it sit for a day.
D. Next day, strain out the extra powder using cheesecloth.
E. Put the oil and beeswax in the double boiler. Heat on low until the wax melts.
F. Pour into small jars or tins right away. Let it cool completely.
G. Use it on sore knees when needed. Keep it somewhere cool so it stays semi-solid.

Special Notes:

- Try adding a few drops of peppermint essential oil for a cooling effect.
- For extra pain relief, warm the salve slightly before applying. Just rub it between your hands for a minute.

2. Soothing Knee Soak

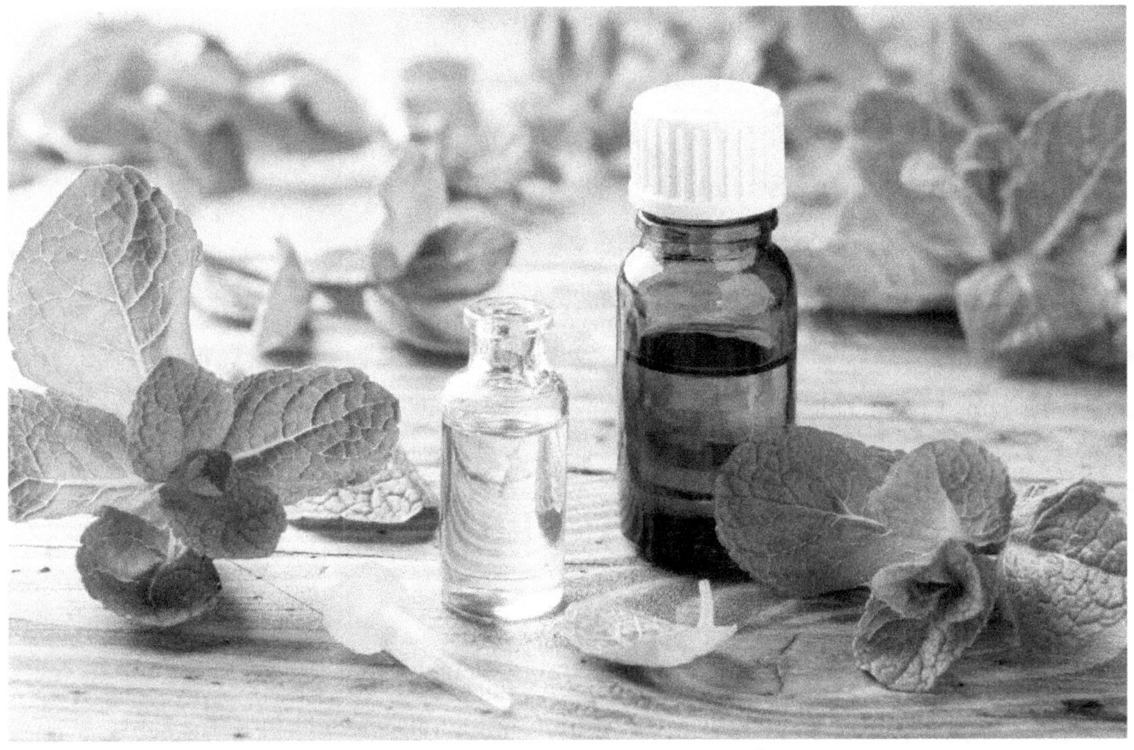

This bath salt mix is a knee pain fighter from your kitchen. It's a simple home remedy that's gaining fans. The mix of Epsom salt and essential oils helps calm sore knees. It's easy to make and feels great. You'll want to soak your knees every day.

Preparation Time: 15 minutes

Serving size: 3 cups (1 cup per bath)

Ingredients:

- 10 drops peppermint essential oil
- 5 drops eucalyptus essential oil
- 5 drops rosemary essential oil
- 5 drops lavender essential oil
- 5 drops cinnamon essential oil
- 2 tablespoons dried lavender flowers
- 1 tablespoon fresh rosemary sprigs
- 1 cup baking soda
- 2 cups Epsom salt

XXXXXXXXXXXXXXXXXXXXXXXXX

Instructions:

A. Get a big bowl. Put the baking soda and Epsom salt in it.
B. Drop in all the essential oils. Mix well until the oils spread out in the salts.
C. Toss in the lavender flowers and rosemary sprigs. Stir them in.
D. Split the mix into 3 jars. Each jar should hold about 1 cup.
E. When you want to use it, pour 1 cup into your bath. Soak your knees for at least 15 minutes.

Special Notes:

- Secret boost: Add a pinch of ginger powder to the mix. It helps with blood flow and might ease pain even more.
- Storage trick: Keep your bath salt mix in a cool, dark place. This helps the essential oils stay strong longer. Your knees will thank you!

3. Soothing Knee Balm

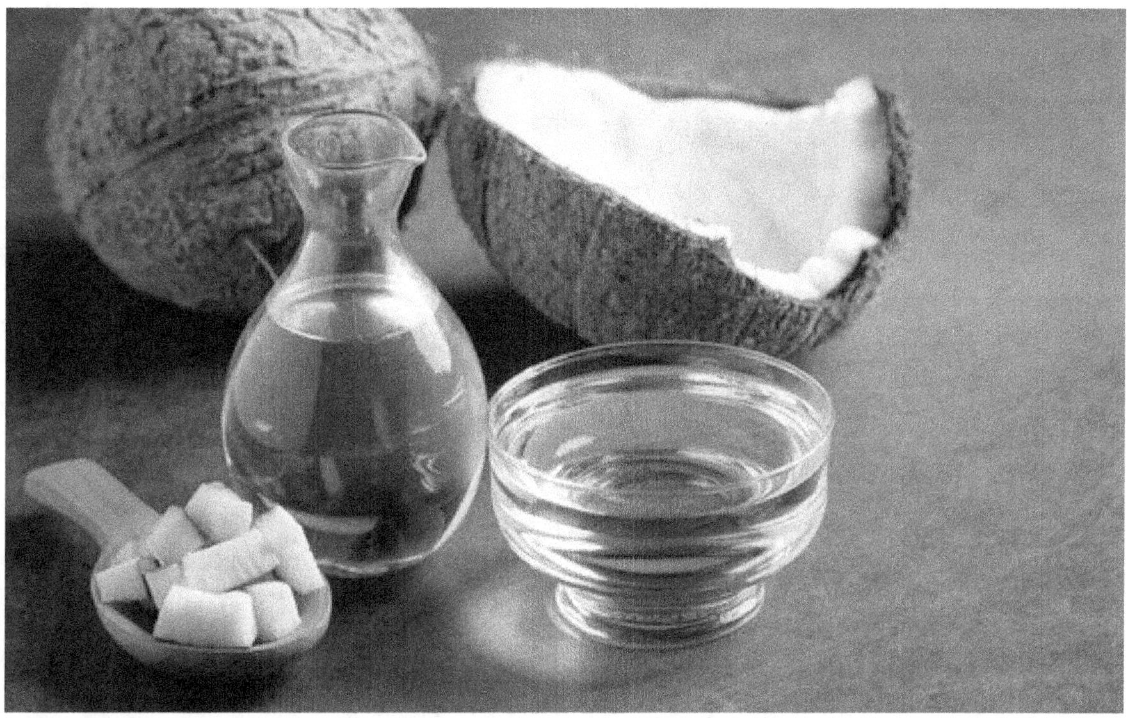

This homemade cream helps ease knee pain so you can move freely. It's quick to make with items you might already have. People love it because it's natural and works fast. The mix of oils smells good too. You'll want to keep a jar handy.

Preparation Time: 10 minutes

Serving size: 20 applications

Ingredients:

- 25 drops myrrh essential oil
- 25 drops frankincense essential oil
- 4 oz unrefined coconut oil
- 10 drops ginger essential oil

XXXXXXXXXXXXXXXXXXXXXXXX

Instructions:

A. Get a small bowl. Put all the oils in it.
B. Stir everything together until it's well mixed.
C. Find a glass jar with a tight lid. Pour the mixture into it.
D. To use, rub the balm on your knees and other sore spots. Do this twice a day.

Special Notes:

- For extra cooling, store the balm in the fridge. The cold feeling can help numb pain.
- Try adding 5 drops of peppermint oil for a tingly, fresh sensation. It might help distract from the pain too.

4. Homemade Mustard Oil Knee Rub

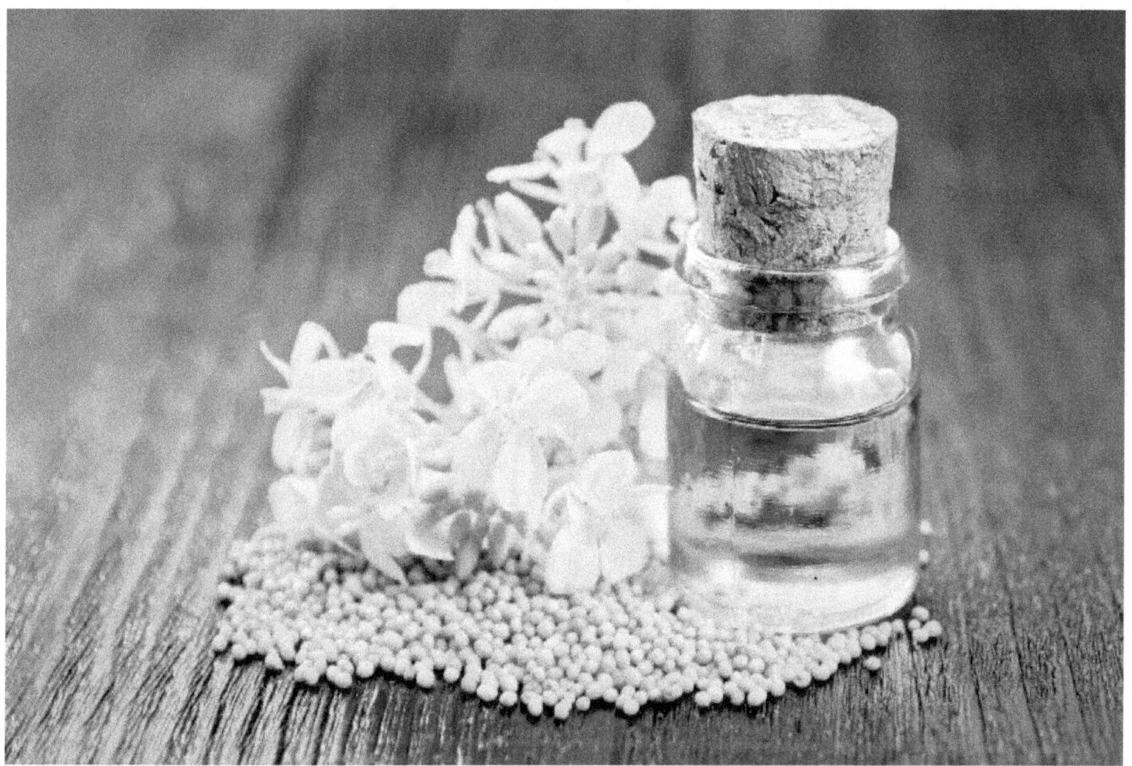

This simple home remedy comes from Asian traditional medicine. It's a quick fix for achy knees using just two ingredients. People love it because it's easy to make and works fast. The mix of mustard oil and caraway seeds creates a warm, soothing feeling that helps with knee pain.

Preparation Time: 12 minutes

Serving size: 1/2 cup

Ingredients:

- 1/2 cup mustard oil
- 1 tablespoon caraway seeds

xxxxxxxxxxxxxxxxxxxxxxxxx

Instructions:

A. Put a small pan on the stove and pour in the mustard oil.
B. Turn the heat to medium-high and wait until the oil gets hot and starts to smoke a little.
C. Toss in the caraway seeds.
D. Right away, turn off the stove.
E. Let the seeds sit in the hot oil. They'll turn black as they cook.
F. Once the oil cools down, it's ready to use. Rub it on your sore knees whenever you need it.

Special Notes:

- For an extra cooling effect, store the oil in the fridge between uses. The contrast between the cool oil and your warm skin can feel really nice.
- If you don't have caraway seeds, you can try using cumin seeds instead. They have similar pain-relieving properties and are often easier to find in regular grocery stores.

5. Knee Soother Roll-On

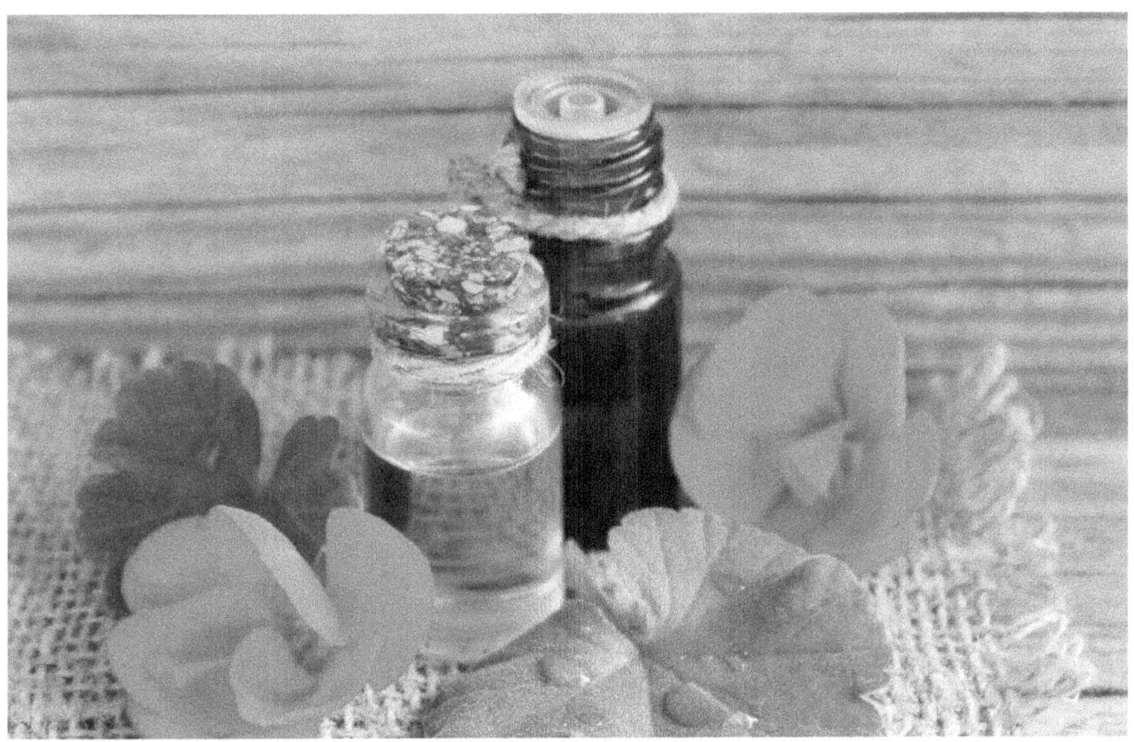

This homemade roll-on is a quick fix for achy knees. It's a simple blend of essential oils that smells nice and helps ease discomfort. People love it because it's easy to make and use. The main ingredients are geranium, lavender, and wintergreen oils mixed with a carrier oil.

Preparation Time: 5 minutes

Serving size: 1 (5ml bottle)

Ingredients:

- 1 (5 ml) glass roller bottle
- 5 drops geranium essential oil
- 5 drops lavender essential oil
- 5 drops wintergreen essential oil
- 4 teaspoons carrier oil (sunflower or olive oil)

xxxxxxxxxxxxxxxxxxxxxxxxx

Instructions:

A. Open your roller bottle.

B. Put in all the essential oils: geranium, lavender, and wintergreen.

C. Add the carrier oil.

D. Close the bottle tight.

E. Shake it well to mix everything.

F. To use, roll it on your sore knee.

G. Gently rub it into your skin.

H. Do this twice a day for best results.

Special Notes:

- Try warming the carrier oil slightly before mixing. This can help the oils blend better and might make the roll-on feel nicer on your skin.
- If you're out of carrier oil, you can use coconut oil instead. It's solid at room temperature, so warm it up a bit first. This swap can add a light, tropical scent to your knee soother.

6. Soothing Knee Balm

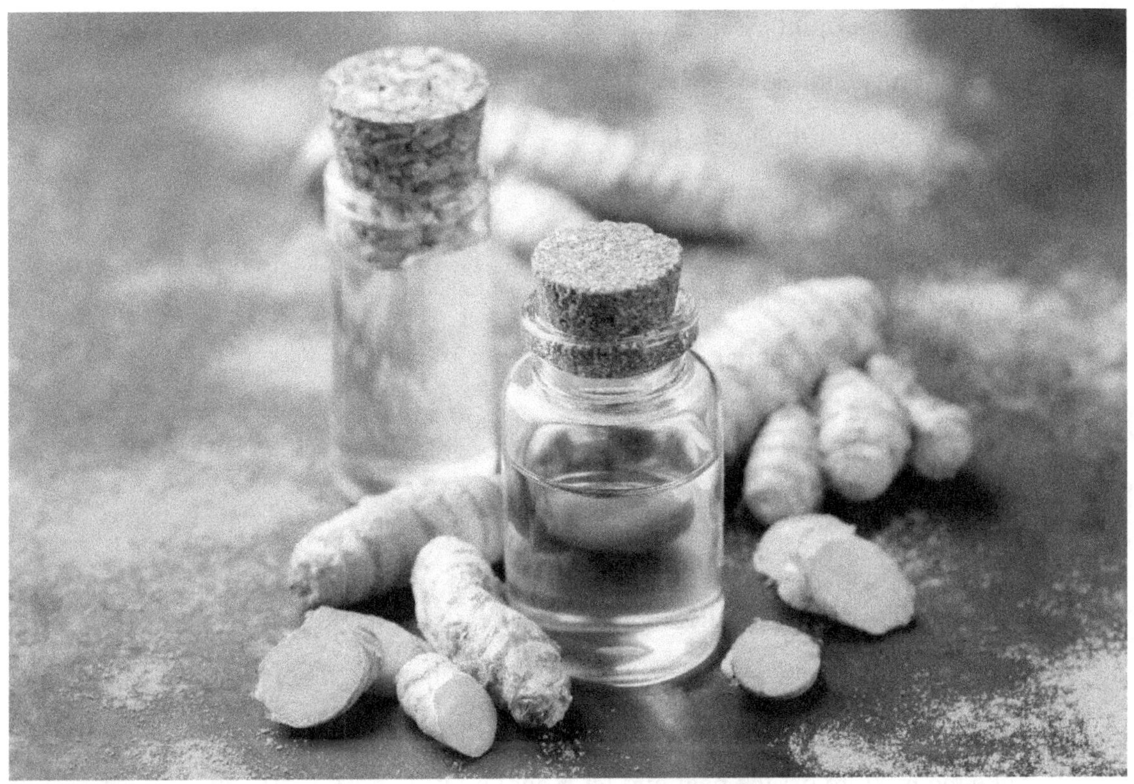

This homemade knee rub is a go-to remedy for many active families. Made with natural ingredients, it's perfect for soothing sore knees after outdoor activities or workouts. The blend of essential oils and nourishing butters makes it a favorite in many households.

Preparation Time: 20 minutes

Serving size: About 3/4 cup

Ingredients:

- 15 drops rosemary essential oil
- 15 drops peppermint essential oil
- 2-3 metal tins with lids
- 1 small mason jar or double boiler
- 1/2 cup unrefined coconut oil
- 1/4 cup shea butter, grated and chopped
- 6 drops turmeric essential oil
- 2 drops lavender essential oil

XXXXXXXXXXXXXXXXXXXXXXXXX

Instructions:

A. Fill a pot with 1 inch of filtered water and heat on medium-low.
B. Place coconut oil and shea butter in a double boiler or mason jar. Set it in the pot.
C. Let the water boil and melt the ingredients. Stir now and then until fully mixed.
D. Take the mixture off the heat and let it cool a bit.
E. Add all the essential oils and mix well.
F. Pour the balm into your tins and let them cool completely.
G. Rub the balm on your knees as needed.
H. Keep the tins in a cool spot in your house.

Special Notes:

- For an extra cooling effect, store the balm in the fridge. The cold temperature will give an added boost to its soothing properties.
- If you're out of shea butter, cocoa butter makes a great substitute. It has similar nourishing properties and will give your balm a lovely chocolate scent.

7. Homemade Knee Warmer

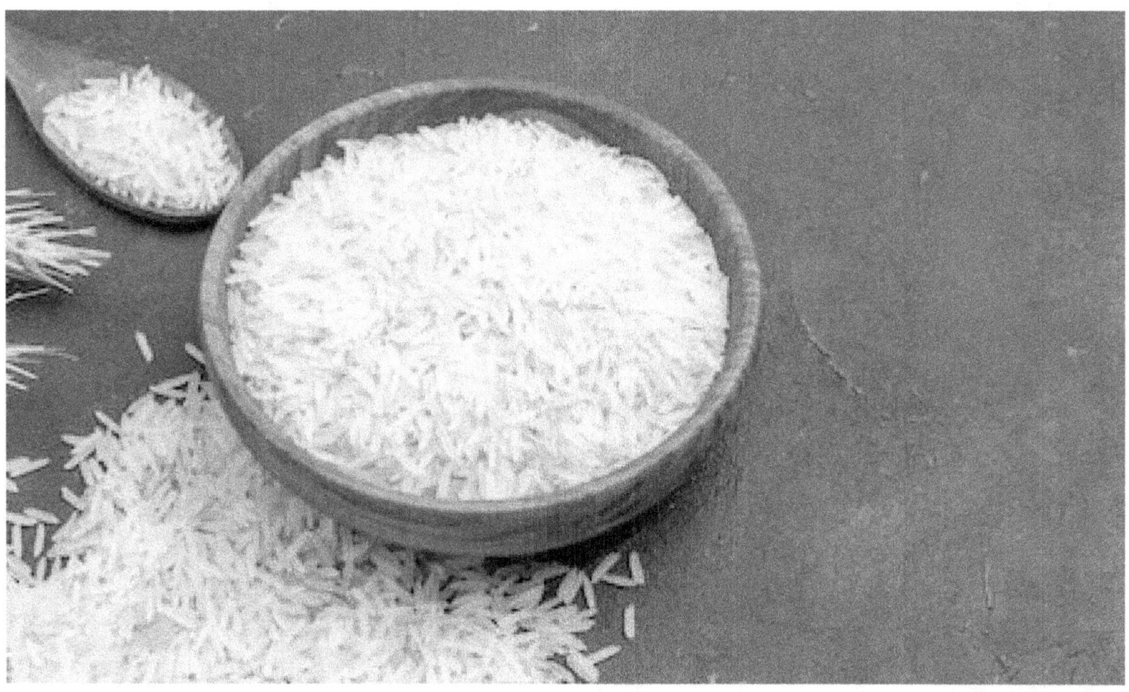

This easy DIY heating pad is perfect for soothing knee pain at home. It's a quick fix using stuff you probably have lying around. People love it because it's cheap, simple, and works great. The main ingredient? Just rice! You'll be amazed at how well this homemade solution helps your achy knees.

Preparation Time: 5-7 minutes

Serving size: 1 heating pad

Ingredients:

- 3 cups uncooked rice
- 1 cotton sock (Do not use synthetic materials)
- Optional: 5 drops lavender essential oil

XXXXXXXXXXXXXXXXXXXXXXXXX

Instructions:

A. Grab your cotton sock. Don't use any other type - cotton's the only safe bet here.
B. Pour the rice into the sock. If you want it to smell nice, add the lavender oil too.
C. Tie the sock tightly so nothing spills out.
D. Pop it in the microwave. Heat it on high for 2-3 minutes.
E. Let it cool a bit. You want it warm, not burning hot.
F. Put it on your knee. The rice will mold to your shape, giving you nice, even heat.
G. Enjoy the warmth for about 30 minutes.

Special Notes:

- Try using jasmine rice for a naturally pleasant scent, even without essential oils.
- Keep a spray bottle handy. A light mist on the sock before heating can add moisture and make the heat last longer.

8. DIY Knee Pain Gel

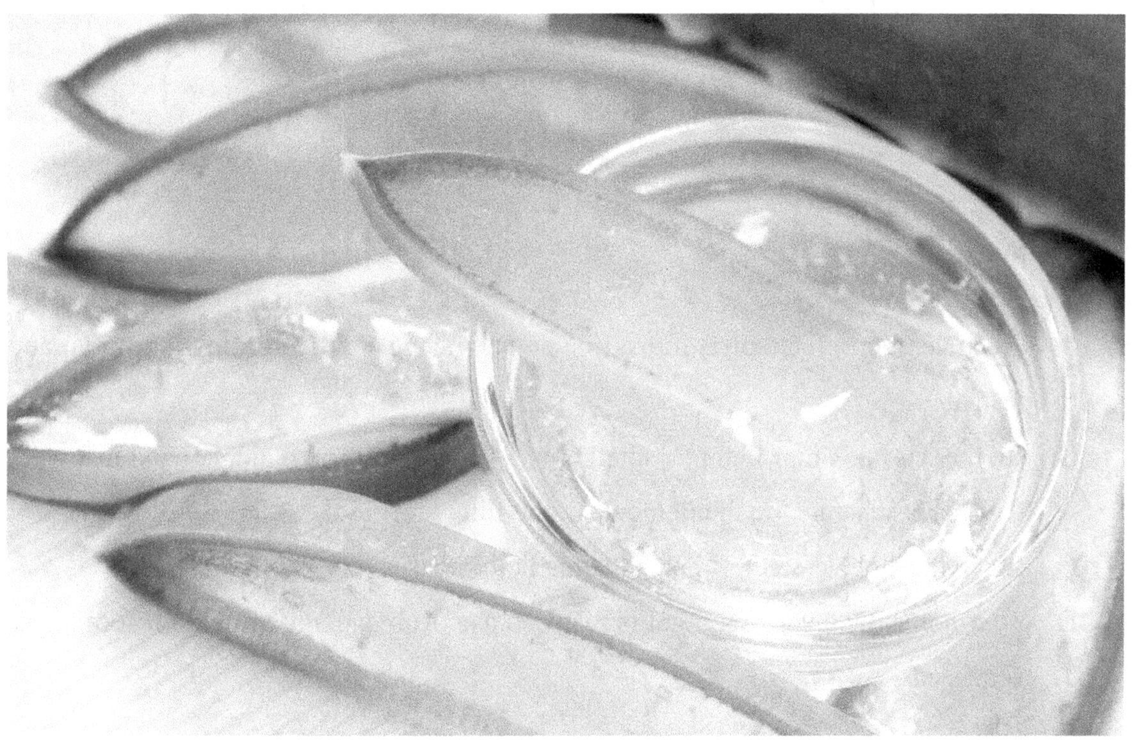

This homemade gel helps with knee pain. It's cheap and easy to make. People like it because it works longer than pills and is safer for your stomach. You can whip it up quickly at home with just a few things from the drugstore.

Preparation Time: 5-10 minutes

Serving size: 1 treatment

Ingredients:

- 2-4 tablets of 325mg ibuprofen, crushed
- 1/4 cup isopropyl alcohol
- 2 tablespoons aloe vera gel

XXXXXXXXXXXXXXXXXXXXXXXXX

Instructions:

A. Crush the ibuprofen tablets into a fine powder using a coffee grinder or mortar and pestle.
B. Put the crushed ibuprofen in a small bowl. Add the isopropyl alcohol and mix well. This helps separate the medicine from the filler stuff in the pills.
C. Stir in the aloe vera gel. It helps the medicine soak into your skin better.
D. Your homemade knee pain gel is ready to use. Rub a small amount on sore knees as needed.

Special Notes:

- For an extra cooling effect, keep your gel in the fridge. The cold can help numb pain too.
- If you're out of aloe vera, try using a bit of coconut oil instead. It also helps the medicine sink in and leaves your skin feeling nice.

9. Orange Knee Soother

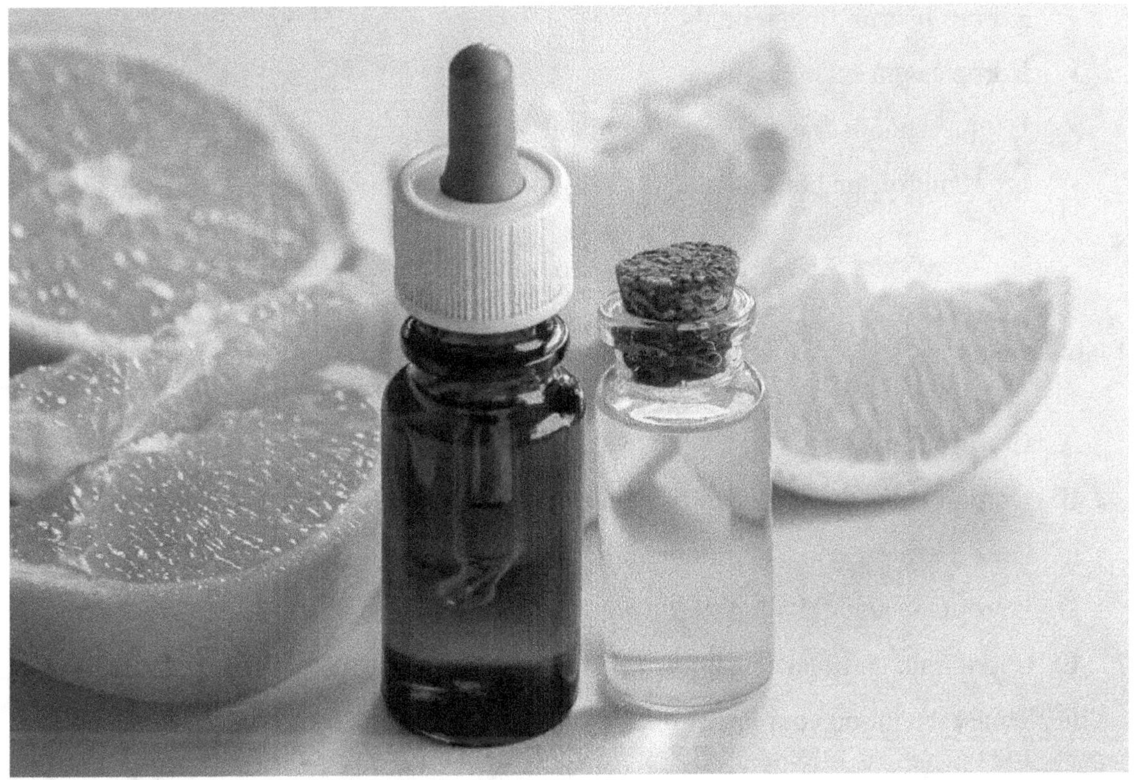

This quick DIY remedy comes from grandma's secret book. It's a hit among folks with achy knees. Orange oil is the star, giving a fresh scent and soothing feel. You'll love how easy it is to make and carry around. It's perfect for those always on the go.

Preparation Time: 5 minutes

Serving size: 1 x 10ml roll-on bottle

Ingredients:

- 2 drops orange essential oil
- 3 drops balsam fir essential oil
- 1 drop cassia essential oil
- 1 3/4 teaspoons fractionated almond oil
- 1 x 10ml roll-on bottle

XXXXXXXXXXXXXXXXXXXXXXXX

Instructions:

A. Grab your roll-on bottle.
B. Drop in the orange, balsam fir, and cassia oils.
C. Give it a good shake to mix the oils.
D. Pour in the almond oil until the bottle's full.
E. Cap it tight and shake again.
F. To use, roll it on your knees or any sore spots.

Special Notes:

- For an extra cooling effect, store your roll-on in the fridge. The cold oil feels great on hot, achy joints.
- If you're out of almond oil, coconut oil works too. It adds a tropical twist to the scent and still soothes your skin.

10. DIY Knee Soother

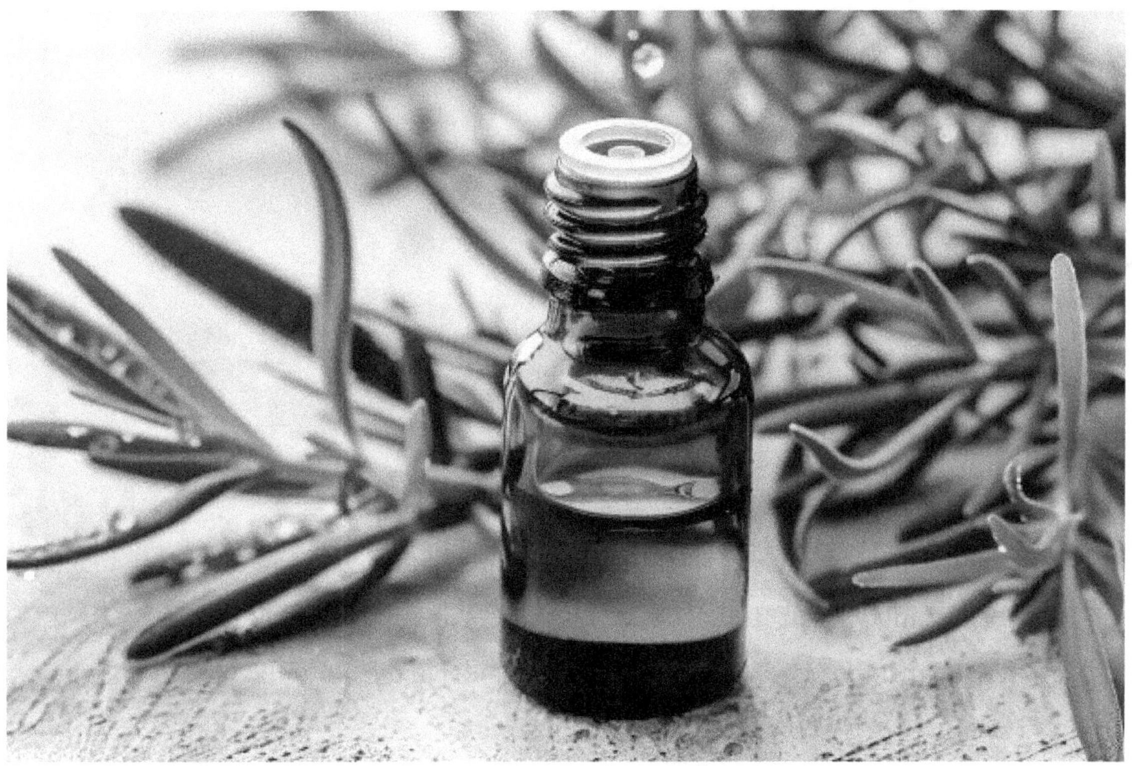

This homemade rub helps ease knee pain with a cooling effect. It's a popular natural remedy that many people swear by. The main ingredients are shea butter, coconut oil, and beeswax, mixed with soothing essential oils. You'll love how easy it is to make and use.

Preparation Time: 20 minutes

Serving size: 9 ounces

Ingredients:

- 3 oz shea butter
- 3 oz coconut oil
- 3 oz beeswax
- 4 to 6 tablespoons menthol crystals
- 20 drops peppermint essential oil
- 10 drops tea tree essential oil
- 2 x 5-oz tins with lids

xxxxxxxxxxxxxxxxxxxxxxxxx

Instructions:

A. Set up a double boiler and melt the shea butter, coconut oil, and beeswax together.
B. Take the mixture off the heat once it's fully melted.
C. Add the menthol crystals, peppermint oil, and tea tree oil to the melted mixture.
D. Stir everything well to combine all ingredients evenly.
E. Carefully pour the mixture into your tins or jars.
F. Let the balm cool and set completely before using.

Special Notes:

- For a smoother application, try whipping the mixture with a hand mixer after it's cooled slightly but before it sets. This creates a lighter, fluffier texture.
- If you want a stronger cooling effect, add a few drops of eucalyptus oil. But be careful - a little goes a long way!

11. Knee Soother Balm

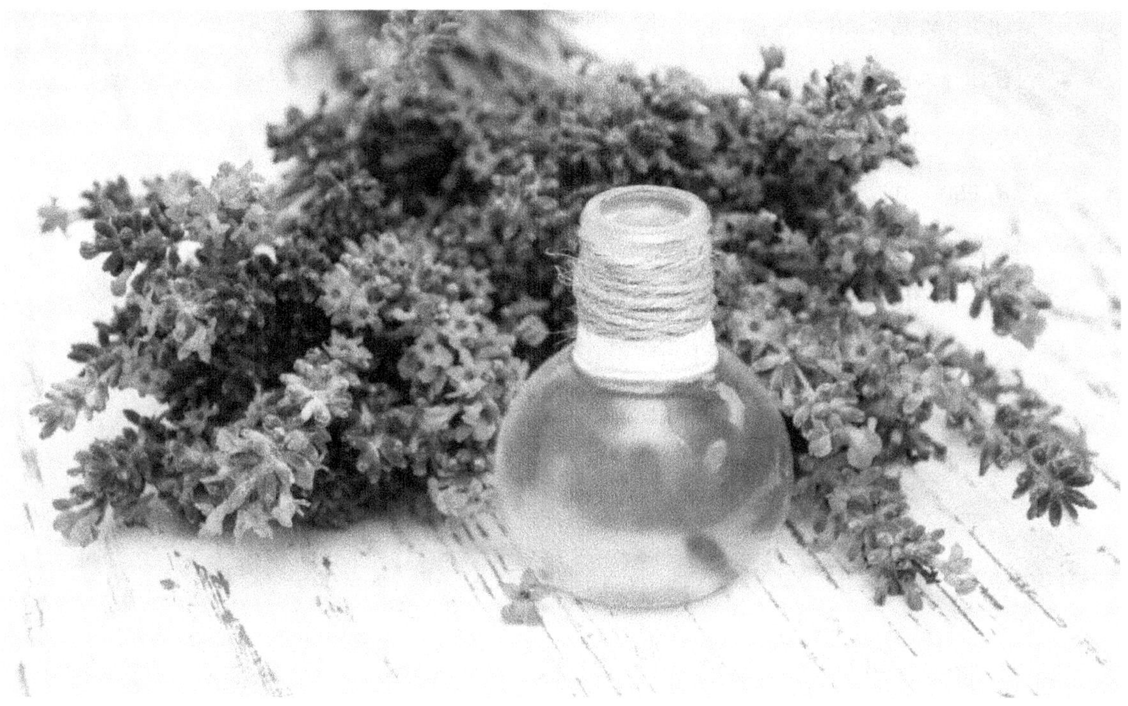

This homemade rub is a natural alternative to store-bought pain relievers. It's easy to make and works wonders for achy knees and other sore spots. The mix of warming and cooling ingredients helps ease discomfort. You'll love how it feels on your skin and how it helps you move more freely.

Preparation Time: 45 minutes

Serving size: 2 ounces

Ingredients:

- 10 drops peppermint essential oil
- 10 drops lavender essential oil
- 10 drops eucalyptus essential oil
- 1/4 cup olive oil or sweet almond oil
- 2 teaspoons cayenne flakes
- 1 tablespoon natural beeswax pellets
- 5 drops clove essential oil
- 5 drops cinnamon essential oil
- 1 (2-oz.) jar or metal tin with lid

XXXXXXXXXXXXXXXXXXXXXXXXX

Instructions:

A. Set up a double boiler with low heat. Pour in the oil.

B. Add cayenne flakes to the oil. Keep heating on very low for 30 minutes. The oil should turn slightly red and smell a bit spicy.

C. Strain the oil through a cheesecloth or sieve. Throw away the cayenne flakes. Put the oil back in the double boiler.

D. Toss in the beeswax. Stir now and then until it melts. Take the mixture off the heat.

E. Mix in all the essential oils gently.

F. Pour the mixture into your jar or tin. Put the lid on right away. Let it cool completely.

G. To use, rub a small amount on your sore knee or other achy spots. Be careful not to touch your eyes or sensitive areas, as the cayenne can sting. Wash your hands well after use.

H. Keep any extra balm in a cool, dark place.

- For an extra cooling effect, try adding a few drops of wintergreen essential oil to the mix. It's great for those who prefer a stronger cooling sensation.
- If you want a smoother texture, try using powdered cayenne instead of flakes. This can make the balm easier to apply and absorb into the skin.

12. Chamomile Knee Soother

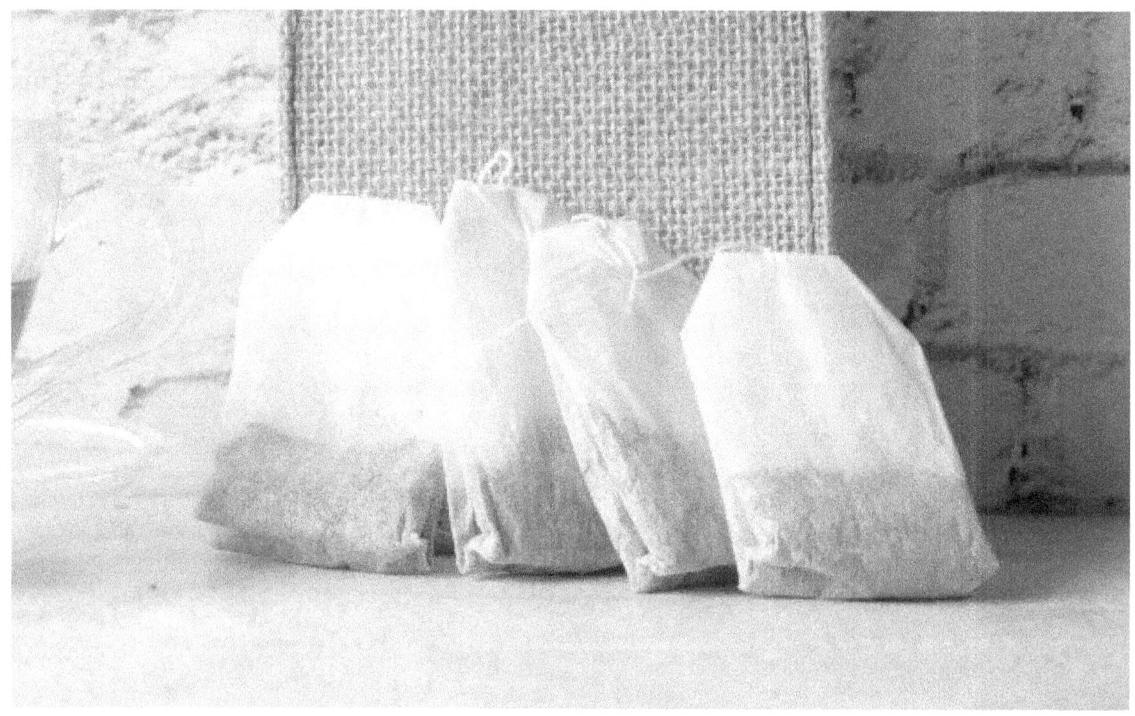

This easy homemade remedy uses chamomile to help soothe knee pain. It's a simple, natural way to care for your knees that people have used for years. You'll only need a few things from your kitchen to make it. It's quick to put together and feels nice on sore knees.

Preparation Time: 30 minutes

Serving size: 1 treatment

Ingredients:

- 4 chamomile tea bags
- 1 cup hot water
- 1 clean cloth (about 12 inches square)

xxxxxxxxxxxxxxxxxxxxxxxxx

Instructions:

A. Make a strong chamomile tea. Put 4 tea bags in 1 cup of hot water.
B. Let the tea sit for 20-25 minutes. Keep it covered while it sits.
C. Take out the tea bags. Squeeze them to get all the tea out.
D. Dip your clean cloth in the tea. It should be warm, not hot.
E. Put the wet cloth on your sore knee.

Special Notes:

- For extra cooling, put the cloth in the fridge for a few minutes before using it.
- If you don't have chamomile tea bags, you can use dried chamomile flowers. Use about 2 tablespoons instead of the tea bags.

13.Soothing Knee Rub

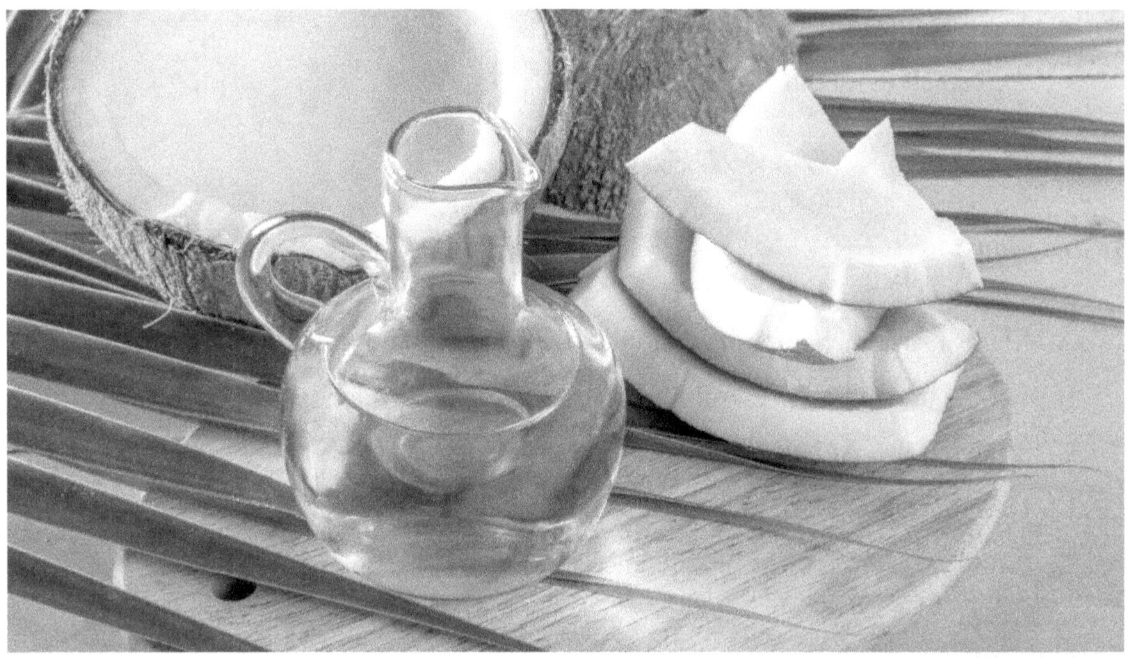

This homemade CBD salve is a quick fix for achy knees. It's easy to make and works better than store-bought creams. People love it because it's natural and doesn't have weird chemicals. You can use it on other sore spots too. It's like a mini massage in a jar.

Preparation Time: 40 minutes

Serving size: 2 ounces

Ingredients:

- 2 ounces coconut oil
- 2 teaspoons beeswax, organic
- 2&1/4 teaspoons shea butter, organic
- 2&1/3 teaspoons CBD oil
- 1 medium glass container for storage

xxxxxxxxxxxxxxxxxxxxxxxx

Instructions:

A. Put the beeswax and shea butter in a double boiler. Heat and stir until they melt together.
B. Add the coconut oil and mix it in.
C. Pour in the CBD oil. Keep stirring until everything is well mixed. Don't let it get too hot.
D. Take the mixture off the heat and let it cool a bit.
E. Pour the slightly cooled mixture into your glass container. Wait for it to cool completely.
F. To use, rub a small amount on your sore knee and massage it in. Keep the rest in a cool, dark place.

Special Notes:

- For extra cooling, add a few drops of peppermint essential oil to the mix. It'll give your knees a nice tingle.
- If you want the salve to smell nice, try adding a bit of lavender oil. It smells good and might help you relax too.

14. Soothing Knee Balm

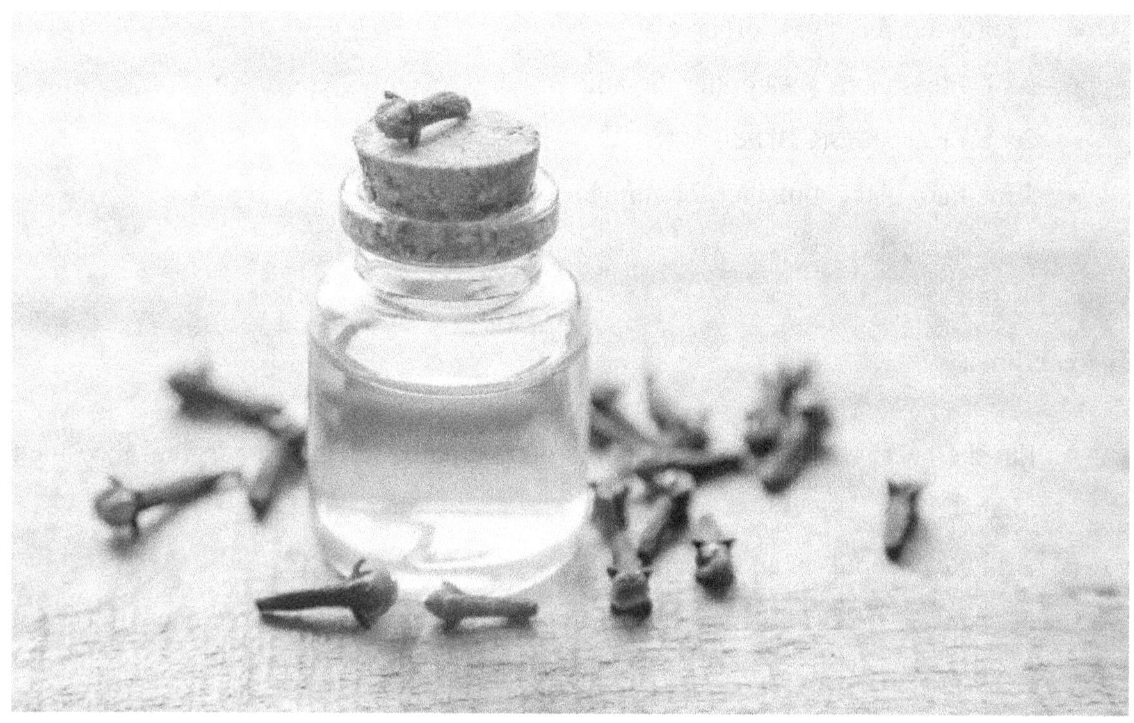

This homemade knee rub is a quick fix for achy joints. It's a simple mix of coconut oil and peppermint, with an optional kick from clove oil. People love it because it's easy to make and works fast. You'll find yourself reaching for it whenever your knees need some TLC.

Preparation Time: 7 minutes

Serving size: 1/2 cup

Ingredients:

- 8 drops peppermint essential oil
- 1/2 cup coconut oil
- Optional: 4 drops clove essential oil

xxxxxxxxxxxxxxxxxxxxxxxxx

Instructions:

A. Put the coconut oil in a microwave-safe container (glass or thick plastic).
B. Zap it in the microwave for 15-20 seconds. The oil should start melting.
C. Give the oil a good stir with a spoon.
D. Drop in the peppermint essential oil.
E. If you want, add the clove essential oil too.
F. Mix everything up really well.
G. Your knee rub is ready! Use it whenever your knees are giving you trouble.

Special Notes:

- Chill factor: For an extra cooling effect, store the balm in the fridge. The cold will give your knees an extra zing when you apply it.
- Scent swap: Not a fan of peppermint? Try using eucalyptus or lavender essential oil instead. They're also great for soothing sore muscles.

15. DIY Knee Pain Balm

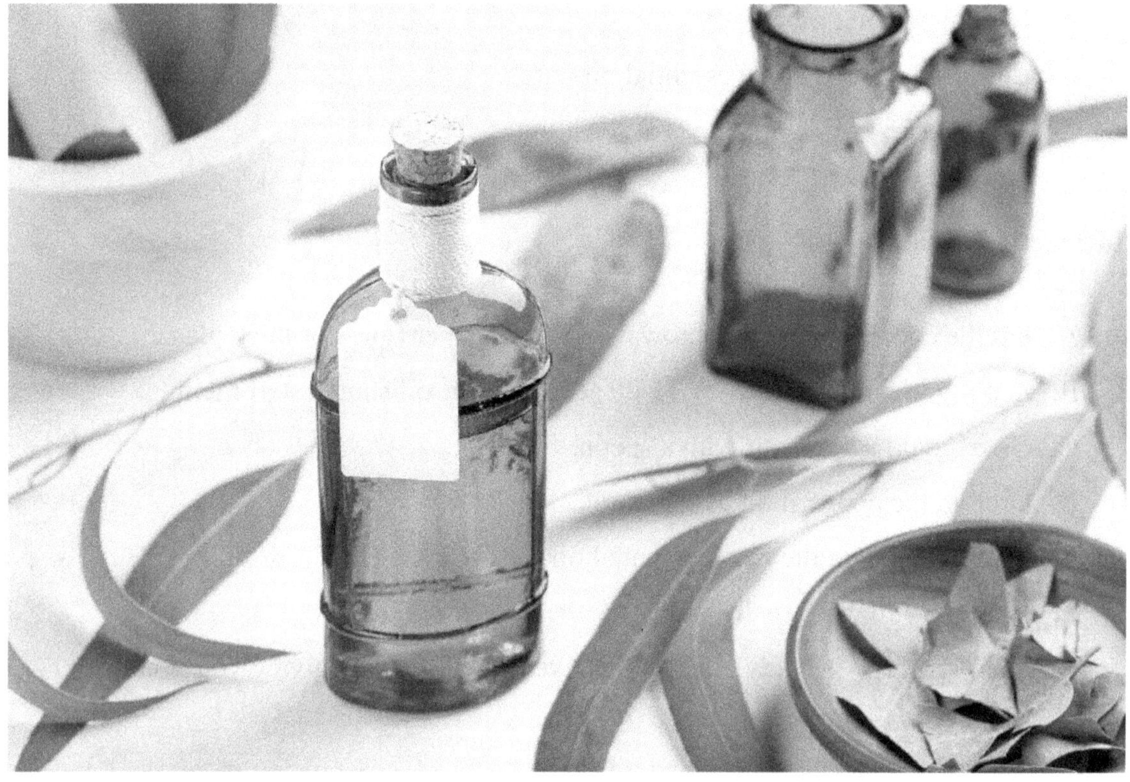

This homemade knee pain balm is a natural remedy that works wonders. It's easy to make and smells great. People love it because it helps with joint pain without the strong menthol scent of store-bought options. The mix of essential oils gives quick relief and a nice aroma.

Preparation Time: 20 minutes

Serving size: Makes about 10 teaspoons

Ingredients:

- 5 drops peppermint essential oil
- 5 drops eucalyptus essential oil
- 4 tablespoons coconut oil
- 5 drops frankincense essential oil
- 5 drops lavender essential oil
- 4 tablespoons natural beeswax
- 1 small glass jar

xxxxxxxxxxxxxxxxxxxxxxxx

Instructions:

A. Put coconut oil and beeswax in a glass bowl.

B. Microwave until everything melts.

C. Take the bowl out of the microwave.

D. Add all the essential oils and mix well.

E. Pour the mix into your glass jar.

F. Put the lid on.

G. Stick it in the fridge to cool faster.

H. Use it whenever you need it.

Special Notes:

- For a smoother texture, try grating the beeswax before melting. It'll mix better with the coconut oil.
- If you want a stronger scent, add an extra drop or two of your favorite essential oil. Just don't go overboard - a little goes a long way!

16. Ginger Knee Soother

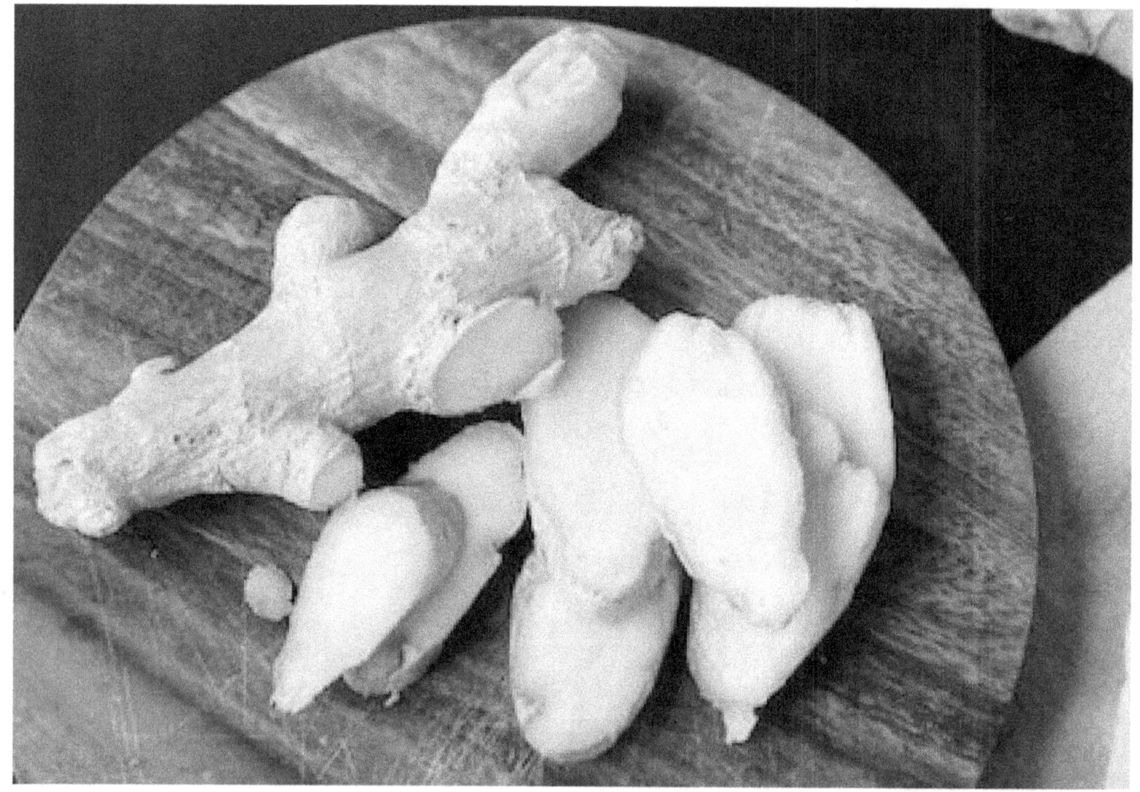

This homemade ginger poultice is a go-to remedy for knee pain. It's popular among those looking for natural relief. The main ingredients are fresh ginger and olive oil. You'll love how easy it is to make and how quickly it can help ease discomfort in your knees, lower back, or wrists.

Preparation Time: 5 minutes

Serving size: 1 treatment

Ingredients:

- 1 piece (3 inches) fresh ginger
- 2-3 tablespoons olive oil, or as needed
- Gauze or ace bandage, enough to wrap around the knee

xxxxxxxxxxxxxxxxxxxxxxxxx

Instructions:

A. Peel the ginger and chop it into very small pieces.
B. Put the chopped ginger in a bowl and add olive oil. Mix well until you get a paste-like consistency.
C. Spread the ginger paste on a piece of gauze or ace bandage.
D. Wrap the gauze or bandage around your knee, making sure the ginger paste is in direct contact with your skin.
E. Leave it on for 10 to 15 minutes.
F. Remove the poultice and gently clean your skin.

Special Notes:

- For extra cooling relief, try adding a few drops of peppermint essential oil to the ginger paste.
- If you don't have fresh ginger, you can use 1-2 teaspoons of dried ginger powder instead. Just make sure to mix it well with the olive oil to avoid any grittiness.

17. Pine Salve for Knee Pain Relief

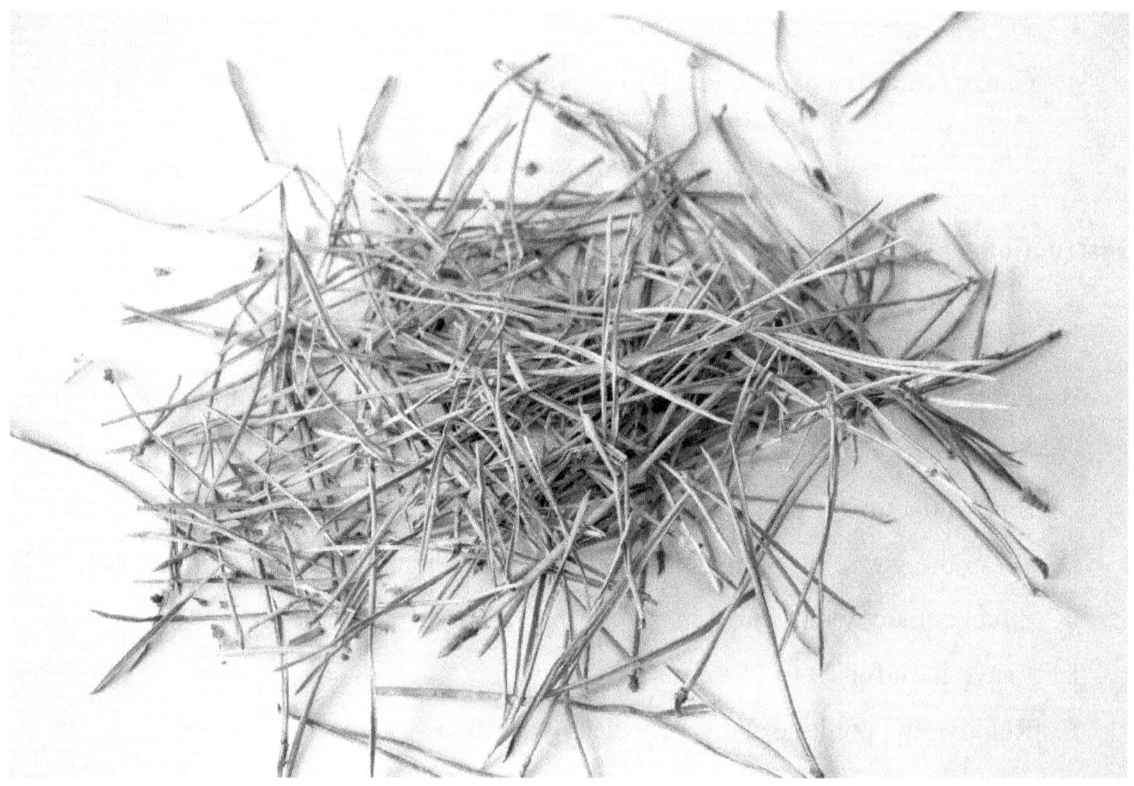

This homemade pine salve is a natural remedy for knee pain. It's easy to make and uses simple ingredients like pine needles and mint. People love it because it's gentle on the skin and smells great. The salve is popular among hikers and older folks who want a natural way to ease their aches.

Preparation Time: 20 minutes

Serving size: 2/3 cup

Ingredients:

- 2 tablespoons dried pine needles, chopped
- 2 tablespoons dried mint leaves, crumbled
- 2/3 cup carrier oil (olive or sunflower oil)
- 5 oz beeswax
- 1/2 - 3/4 teaspoons peppermint essential oil

xxxxxxxxxxxxxxxxxxxxxxxxx

Instructions:

A. Soak the pine needles and mint leaves in the carrier oil until the oil takes on their scent. Then, strain the oil to remove the plant bits.

B. Put 1/2 cup of the scented oil and the beeswax in a glass jar.

C. Place the jar in a pot with 1-2 inches of water. Heat on medium-low until the beeswax melts.

D. Take the jar off the heat. Add the peppermint essential oil and mix well.

E. Pour the mixture into small containers.

F. To use, rub a small amount on sore knees or other achy spots.

Special Notes:

- For a stronger scent, add a drop of eucalyptus oil. It pairs well with pine and can help clear your sinuses too.
- If you don't have pine needles, you can use rosemary instead. It has similar pain-relieving properties and smells great with mint.

18. Spicy Knee Soother

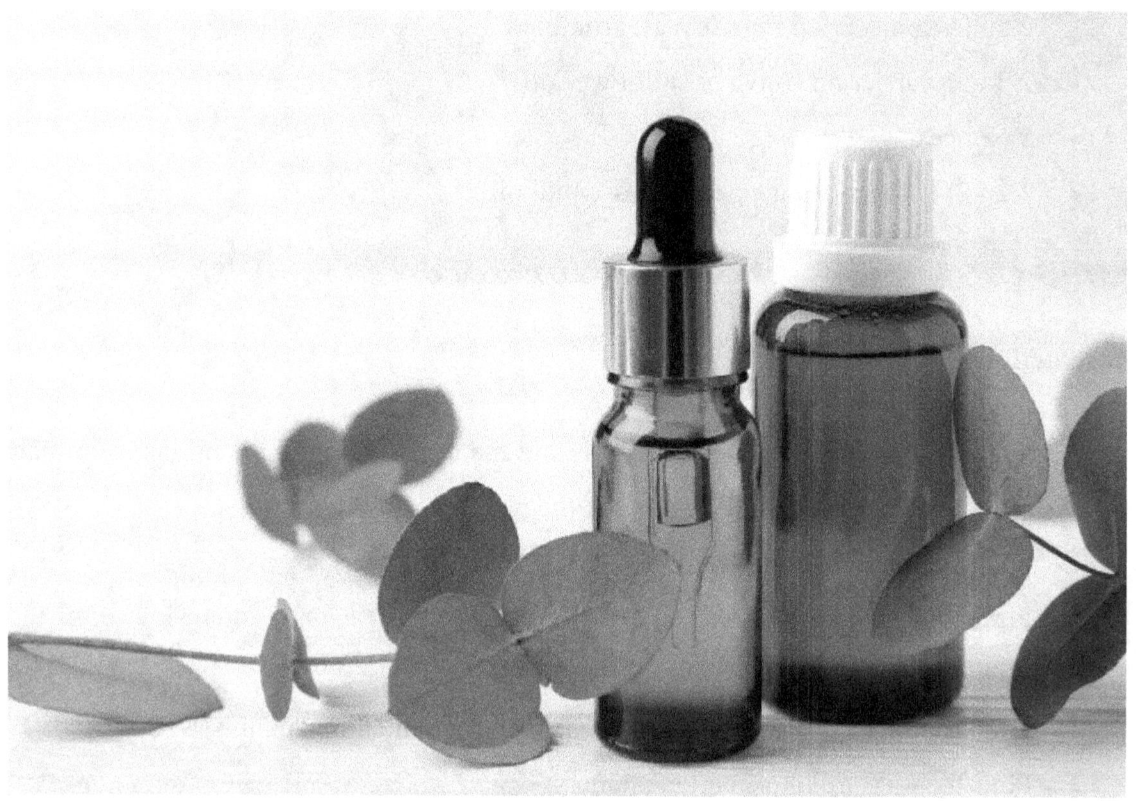

This homemade rub is a favorite among outdoor workers. It's great for easing knee pain. The cayenne pepper boosts blood flow, which helps reduce swelling and soreness. It's easy to make and really works. You'll love how it warms and soothes your achy knees.

Preparation Time: 1 hour 15 minutes

Serving size: 1 cup

Ingredients:

- 50 drops peppermint essential oil
- 50 drops eucalyptus essential oil
- 40 drops copaiba essential oil
- 1/2 cup coconut oil
- 2 tablespoons cayenne pepper
- 2 tablespoons grated beeswax
- 1/2 cup shea butter
- Optional: 30 drops rosemary essential oil

xxxxxxxxxxxxxxxxxxxxxxxxx

Instructions:

A. Set up a double boiler. If you don't have one, use two pots that fit inside each other.

B. Mix coconut oil and cayenne pepper in the top pot. Warm it up a bit.

C. Stir the mix, then let it sit for 30 minutes.

D. Warm it again, then set it aside to let the cayenne soak in more.

E. Strain the oil through cheesecloth into a 1/4 cup measure. Top up with extra coconut oil if needed.

F. In the double boiler, melt shea butter and beeswax together.

G. Add your cayenne oil to this mix. Put in half of each essential oil.

H. Pour into a container with a tight lid.

I. Repeat steps 5-8 with the remaining 1/4 cup of oil and essential oils.

J. Use on sore knees as needed. Do a skin test first to check for any reactions.

K. Keep in a cool, dry spot.

Special Notes:

- For extra kick, add a pinch of ginger powder to the cayenne mix. It gives an extra warming boost.
- Try using cocoa butter instead of shea butter for a chocolatey scent that pairs well with the spicy cayenne.

19. DIY Pain-Be-Gone Sticks

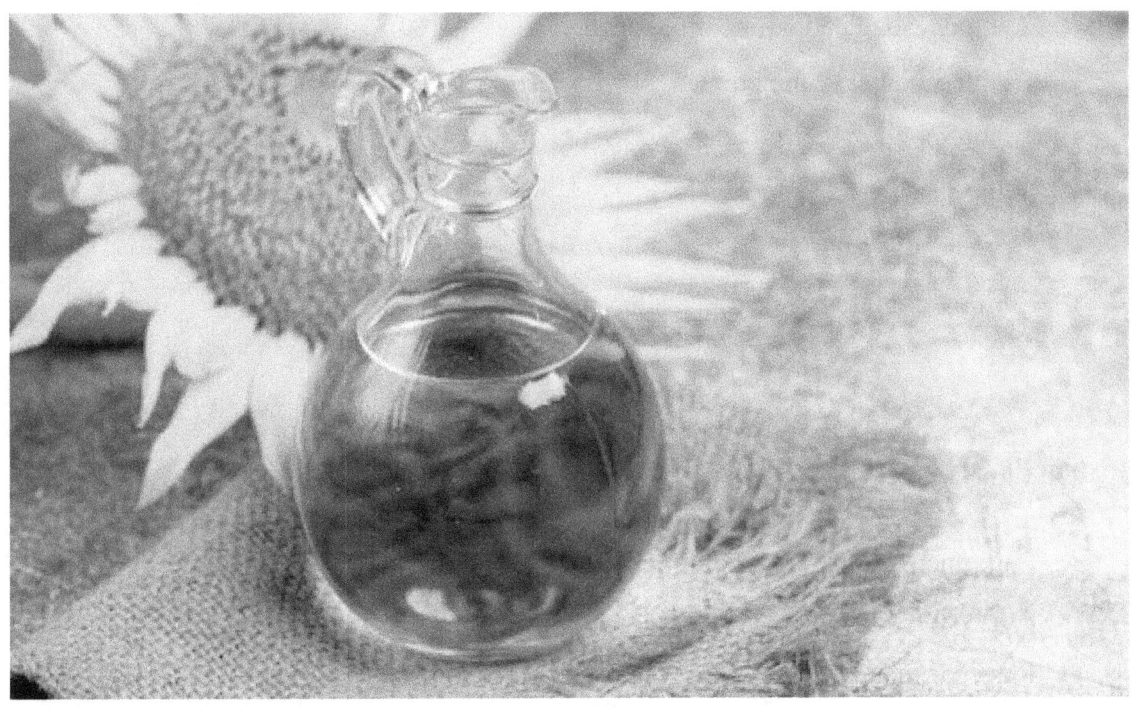

This homemade balm helps ease knee pain. It's easy to make and apply. The recipe comes from old remedies. People like it because it works fast. It uses natural stuff like arnica and cayenne. You'll love how it soothes your sore knees.

Preparation Time: 2 hours 30 minutes

Serving size: Makes 4 ounces (2 x 2-ounce sticks)

Ingredients:

- 2 tablespoons dried arnica flowers
- 2 empty 2-oz deodorant containers
- 1 tablespoon cayenne powder
- 1 tablespoon ginger powder
- 3 oz beeswax
- 7 oz shea butter
- Sunflower oil (as needed)

XXXXXXXXXXXXXXXXXXXXXXXXX

Instructions:

A. Put arnica, cayenne, and ginger in a glass jar.
B. Add sunflower oil to cover. Mix well.
C. Place jar in a pot with warm water. Heat on low for 1-2 hours.
D. Strain the oil. Throw away the bits left in the strainer.
E. Mix beeswax, shea butter, and the oil in a clean glass jar.
F. Put this jar in a pot with warm water. Heat until everything melts.
G. Let it cool a bit, then pour into deodorant containers.
H. Use on sore knees. Keep away from eyes.

Special Notes:

- For extra kick, add a few drops of peppermint oil. It gives a cool feeling and smells nice.
- If you don't have sunflower oil, coconut oil works too. It's good for skin and melts easily.

20. Knee-Soothing Herbal Rub

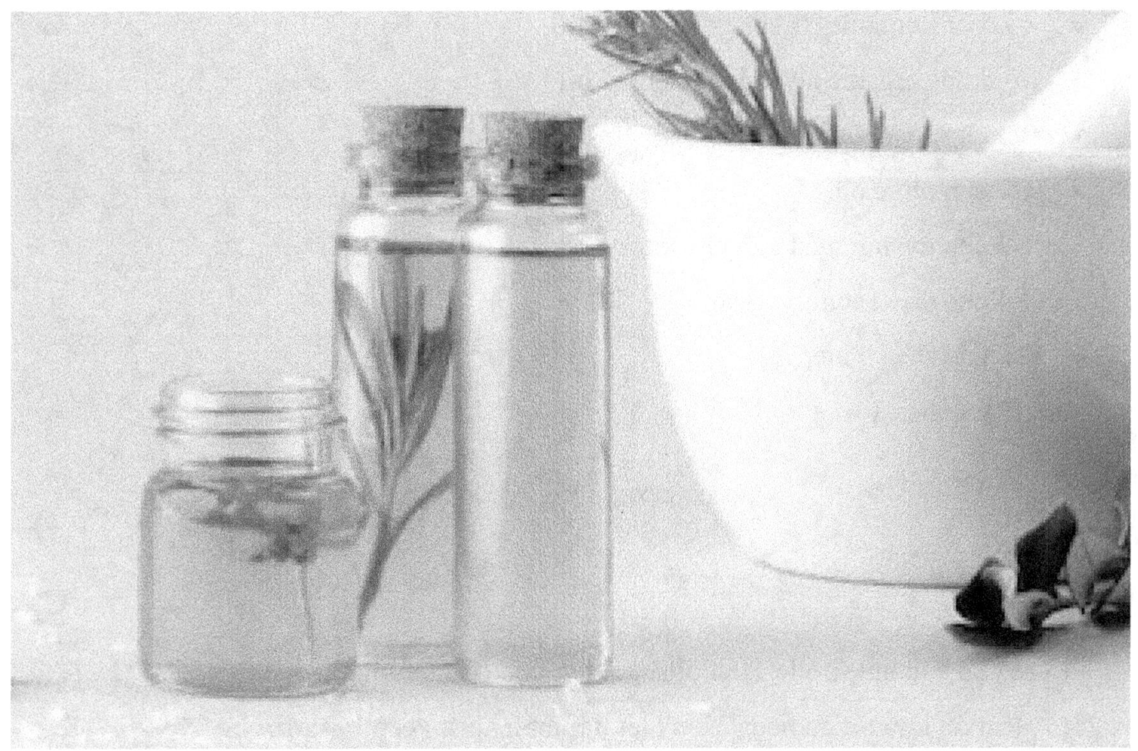

This homemade remedy comes from old folk medicine. It's a mix of herbs and oils that many people use to ease sore knees. The main ingredients are comfrey and ginger. It's easy to make and might help you feel better. Give it a try if you're looking for a natural option.

Preparation Time: 25 minutes

Serving size: 2 1/2 cups

Ingredients:

- 40 drops organic cypress essential oil
- 40 drops organic rosemary essential oil
- 40 drops organic lavender essential oil
- 2/3 cup coconut oil
- 1/2 cup olive oil
- 1/2 cup fresh grated ginger root
- 1/4 cup dried comfrey leaf
- 1/2 cup shea butter
- 1/2 cup beeswax

XXXXXXXXXXXXXXXXXXXXXXXXX

Instructions:

A. Set up a double boiler. Put oils, ginger, and comfrey in the top part.

B. Heat on low for an hour. Don't let it bubble, just keep it warm.

C. Strain the mix through a sieve or cheesecloth.

D. Add beeswax and shea butter to the oil. Stir until they melt. Turn up the heat a bit if needed.

E. Let the mix cool down.

F. Add the essential oils and mix well.

G. Put in a jar and keep in a cool, dry spot.

H. Use on your knees when they hurt.

Special Notes:

- For extra cooling, store the rub in the fridge. It feels great on hot, achy joints.
- Try adding a few drops of peppermint oil for a nice tingle. Start with just a little to see how you like it.

21. Knee Pain DIY Herbal Oil

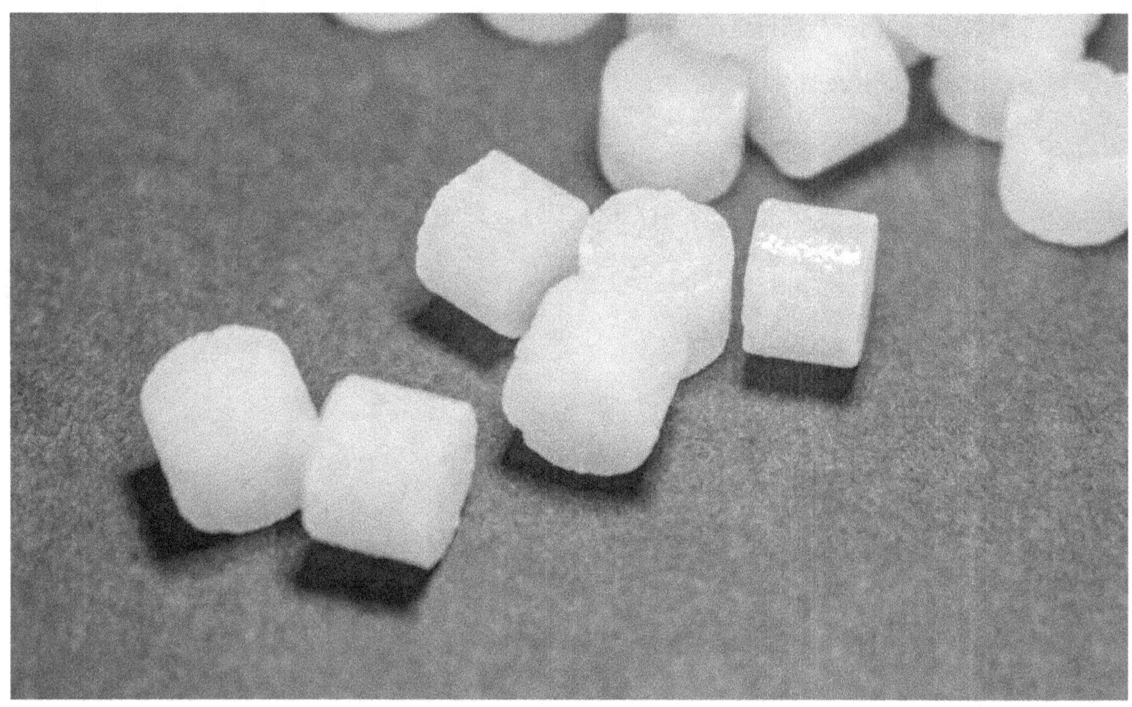

This homemade oil blend comes straight from India's traditional medicine. It's a mix of common spices and herbs that people have used for ages to help with knee pain. If your knees are giving you trouble, this might be worth a try. It's easy to make and uses stuff you can find in most kitchens.

Preparation Time: 45 minutes + overnight sitting

Serving size: 2 cups

Ingredients:

- 20 crushed camphor tablets
- 5 tablespoons aloe vera gel
- 5 cinnamon sticks (2 inches each)
- 1 cup sesame oil
- 1 cup mustard oil
- 1/2 cup chopped or sliced garlic cloves
- 1 tablespoon whole cloves
- 2 tablespoons black sesame seeds
- 3 tablespoons carom seeds
- 2 tablespoons fenugreek seeds
- Optional: 1 tablespoon turmeric powder

xxxxxxxxxxxxxxxxxxxxxxxx

Instructions:

A. Put the sesame and mustard oils in a pan. Turn the heat to medium.

B. Toss in all the other stuff, except the camphor and turmeric.

C. Turn the heat down low. Let it cook until the garlic turns black and crispy.

D. Take the pan off the heat. Now add the camphor and turmeric if you're using it.

E. Let the mix sit overnight. This gives the oil time to soak up all the good stuff from the herbs and spices.

F. The next day, strain the oil. Pour it into a big glass jar that can hold at least 2 cups.

G. To use, rub some on your knees and massage it gently.

Special Notes:

- For an extra cooling effect, keep the oil in the fridge. The cold oil can feel nice on sore knees.
- If you're not a fan of the strong smell, add a few drops of lavender oil. It'll make it smell nicer without messing up the recipe.

22. Knee Soother Salve

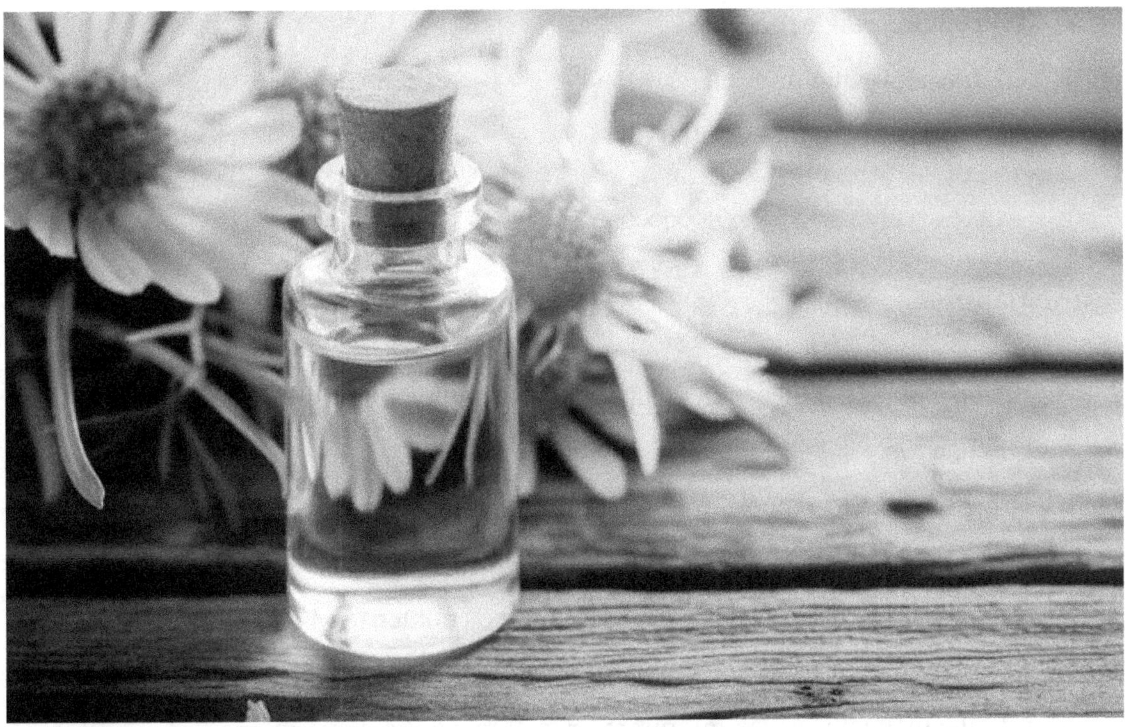

This homemade salve is a must-have for anyone with achy knees. It's a simple blend of natural ingredients that work together to ease pain and swelling. People love it because it's easy to make and really helps. You'll find yourself reaching for it often after a long day or tough workout.

Preparation Time: 1 hour 10 minutes

Serving size: 8 ounces (4 x 2-ounce tins)

Ingredients:

- 3/4 cup arnica oil
- 1/4 cup beeswax pellets
- 1/2 teaspoon vitamin E oil
- 20 drops peppermint essential oil

xxxxxxxxxxxxxxxxxxxxxxxx

Instructions:

A. Set up a double boiler with 2 cups of water in the bottom pot. Put a heat-safe glass bowl on top.
B. Bring the water to a boil. Add the arnica oil and beeswax pellets to the glass bowl. Stir for about 5 minutes until the beeswax melts completely.
C. Take the bowl off the heat. Let it cool on the counter for a few minutes.
D. Mix the vitamin E oil and peppermint essential oil in a small container. Pour this into the melted beeswax mixture. Stir well to combine everything.
E. Pour the mixture into a measuring cup, then divide it evenly among four 2-ounce tins.
F. Let the salve cool and harden fully. Store the tins in a cool place when not using.

Special Notes:

- For an extra cooling effect, try adding a few drops of eucalyptus oil along with the peppermint.
- If you want a firmer salve, increase the beeswax slightly. For a softer texture, use a bit less. Experiment to find your perfect consistency.

23. Knee Soothing Herbal Brew

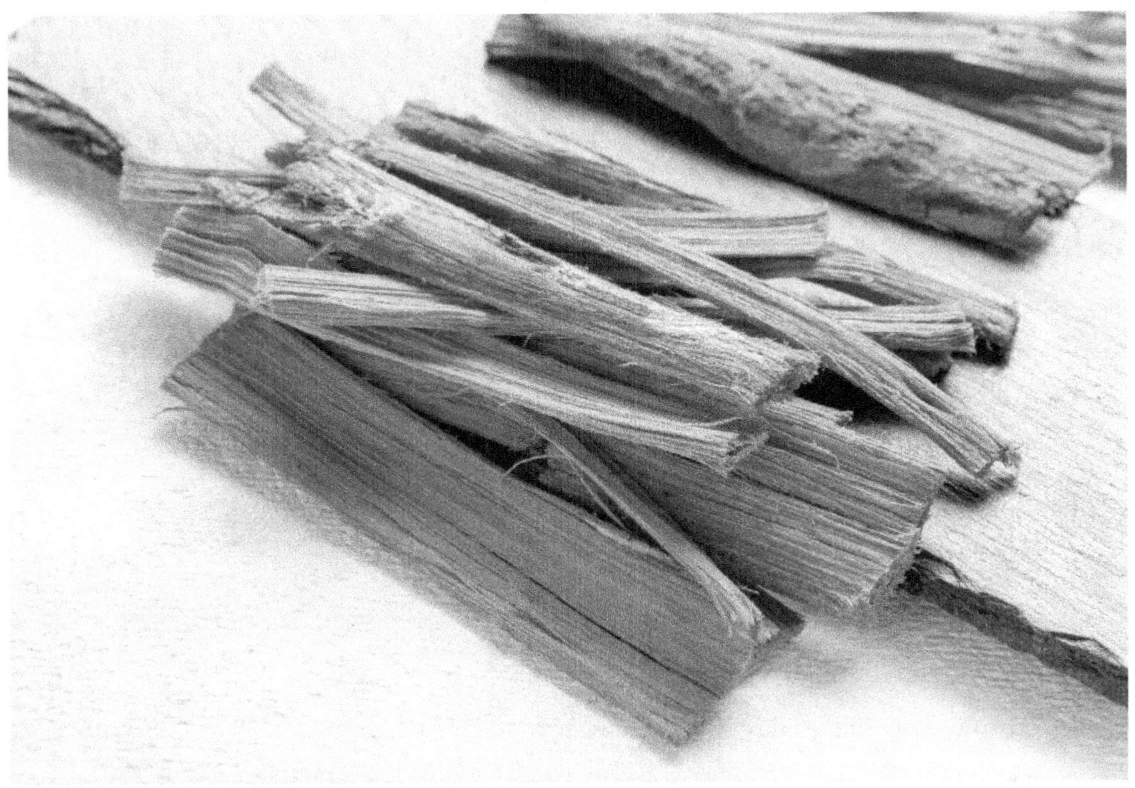

This tea comes from old healing traditions. It's getting more popular as people look for natural ways to feel better. Cat's claw and peony are the stars here. They work together to help your knees feel less sore. It's easy to make and tastes pretty good too. You'll like how it makes your knees feel after drinking it for a while.

Preparation Time: 45 minutes

Serving size: 4 cups

Ingredients:

- 4 cups filtered water
- 1 oz cat's claw bark
- 2 oz peony leaves

XXXXXXXXXXXXXXXXXXXXXXXXX

Instructions:

A. Put the cat's claw bark in a pot.

B. Add the filtered water to cover the bark.

C. Heat it up on low.

D. Let it simmer for 30 minutes.

E. Add the peony leaves.

F. Keep simmering for 10 more minutes.

G. Pour the tea through a strainer.

H. Throw away the used herbs.

I. Drink this tea once or twice a day to help your knees feel better.

Special Notes:

- Try adding a cinnamon stick while brewing for a warm, spicy twist.
- If you find the taste too strong, mix in a spoonful of honey. It'll make it sweeter and add some extra health perks.

24. Juniper Knee Balm

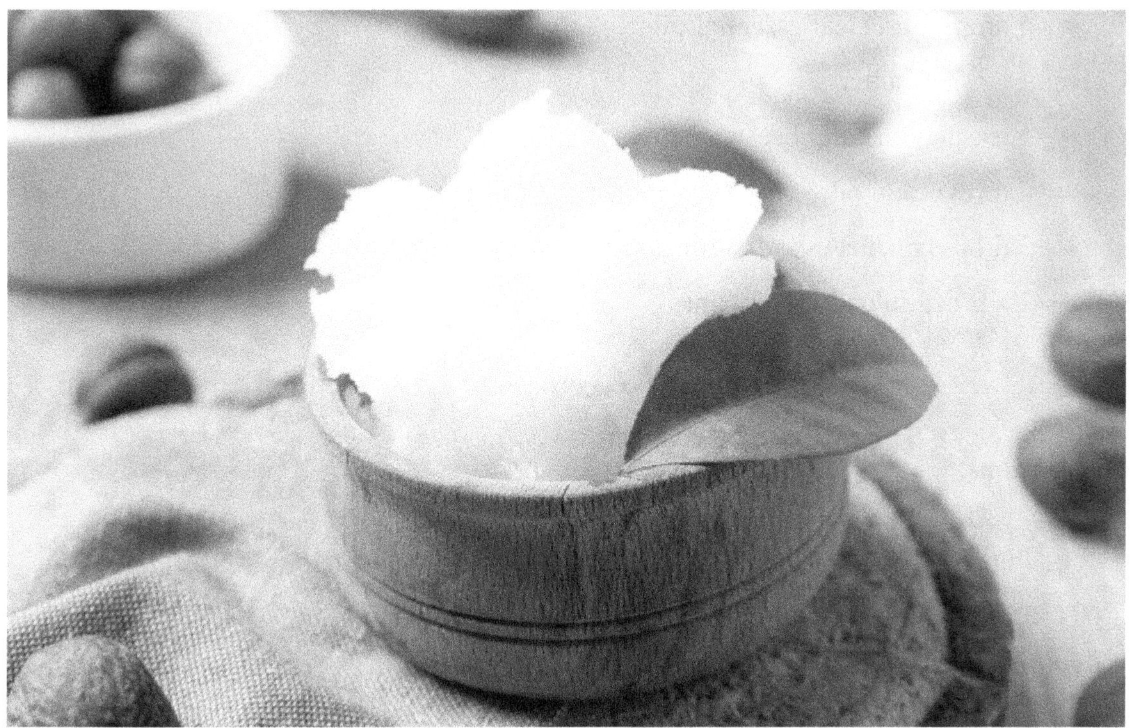

This homemade balm uses juniper berry oil to ease sore knees. It's a quick and easy remedy that smells like a forest. People love it because it works fast and feels nice on the skin. You can make it at home with just a few ingredients.

Preparation Time: 35 minutes

Serving size: 2 oz.

Ingredients:

- 10 drops juniper berry essential oil
- 5 drops laurel leaf essential oil
- 1 oz shea butter
- 1 teaspoon natural beeswax
- 5 oz avocado oil
- 3 drops copaiba essential oil
- 1 x 2-oz. tin or 2 x 1-oz. tins

XXXXXXXXXXXXXXXXXXXXXXXX

Instructions:

A. Put some water in a small pan. Place a glass measuring cup in it. Heat on low.
B. Put the beeswax in the cup. Let it melt.
C. Add shea butter and avocado oil. Stir until everything melts. Let it cool a bit.
D. Put in the essential oils. Mix well.
E. Pour into your tin(s). Let it cool some more, then put the lids on.
F. To use, rub a small amount on your knee. Keep the balm in a cool, dark place.

Special Notes:

- Try adding a drop of peppermint oil for a cooling effect.
- For extra smoothness, whip the mixture with a hand mixer before it sets completely.

25. Turmeric Milk Elixir

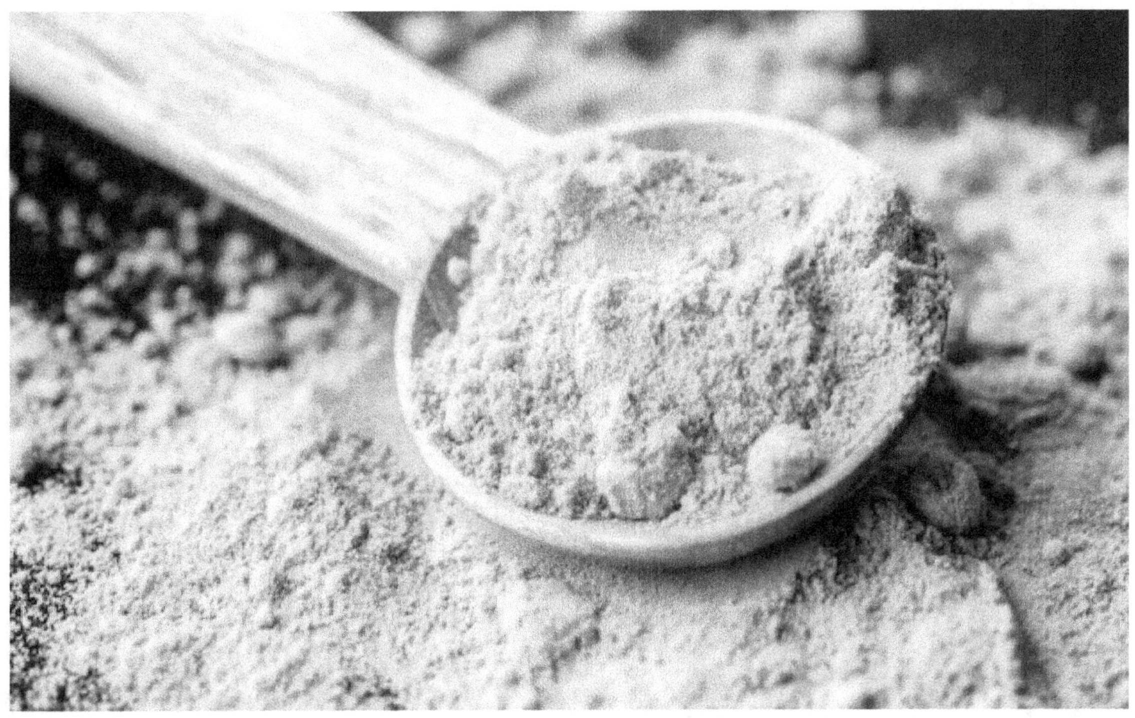

This healing drink comes from India. It's getting popular worldwide for its knee pain relief. The star is turmeric, mixed with milk and spices. It's warm, comforting, and might just be your new favorite bedtime drink. People love it for its gentle, earthy taste and potential health perks.

Preparation Time: 10 minutes

Serving size: 1 cup

Ingredients:

- 1 cup low-fat milk
- 1 teaspoon ground turmeric
- 1/4-inch fresh ginger, grated
- 1 pinch black pepper
- Honey to taste

XXXXXXXXXXXXXXXXXXXXXXXXX

Instructions:

A. Pour the milk into a small pot.

B. Add the turmeric, grated ginger, and black pepper.

C. Heat the mixture on medium-low, stirring often.

D. Let it simmer for about 5 minutes until it's warm and the flavors mix.

E. Turn off the heat.

F. Stir in some honey until it tastes good to you.

G. Pour into a mug and drink while it's warm.

Special Notes:

- For a richer taste, try using coconut milk instead of regular milk. It adds a tropical twist and some people find it easier to digest.
- If you want an extra boost, add a small cinnamon stick while heating. It gives a nice aroma and might help with inflammation too.

26. Knee Soother Cream

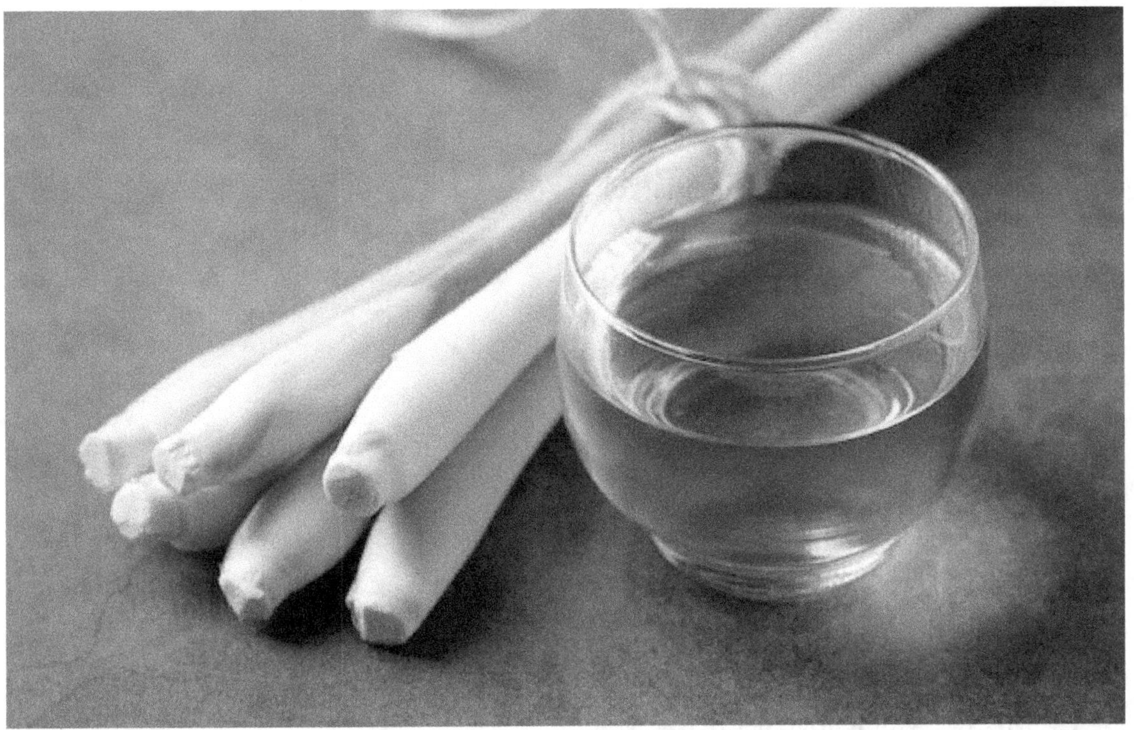

This homemade cream is a lifesaver for achy knees. It's quick to make and works like magic. People love it because it uses natural ingredients and essential oils. You'll feel the difference right away. It's perfect for anyone with knee troubles, whether from sports, getting older, or just everyday life.

Preparation Time: 15 minutes

Serving size: 8 ounces

Ingredients:

- 35 drops copaiba essential oil
- 35 drops peppermint essential oil
- 20 drops wintergreen essential oil
- 20 drops lemongrass essential oil
- 20 drops frankincense essential oil
- 10 drops myrrh essential oil
- 1 cup coconut oil
- 2 x 4 oz jars for storing and using

xxxxxxxxxxxxxxxxxxxxxxxx

Instructions:

A. Put the coconut oil in a medium bowl. Beat it until it's light and fluffy.
B. Add all the essential oils to the whipped coconut oil.
C. Mix everything together really well.
D. Scoop the mixture into your jars.
E. Use on your knees whenever you need it.

Special Notes:

- For an extra cooling effect, keep one jar in the fridge. The cold cream feels great on hot, swollen knees.
- If you want a smoother cream, melt the coconut oil first, mix in the oils, then let it cool and whip it up. This makes it easier to spread.

27. Fenugreek Knee Soother

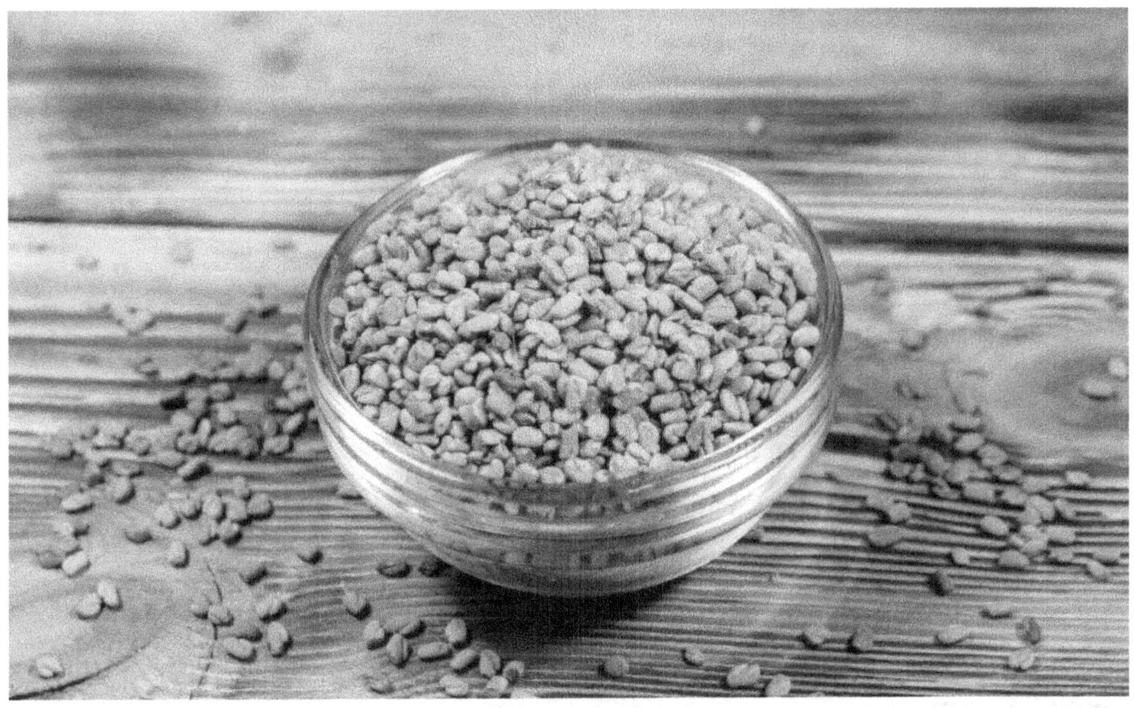

This old Indian remedy is a hit for knee pain. People love it because it's easy to make and works well. Fenugreek seeds are the star here. They help with swelling and pain. You'll like how simple it is to use and how it can make your knees feel better.

Preparation Time: 8 hours (overnight soaking)

Serving size: 1 treatment

Ingredients:

- 2 tablespoons fenugreek seeds
- 1 cup filtered water

XXXXXXXXXXXXXXXXXXXXXXXXXX

Instructions:

A. Put 2 tablespoons of fenugreek seeds in a bowl.

B. Add 1 cup of filtered water to cover the seeds.

C. Let the seeds soak in the water overnight or for about 8 hours.

D. In the morning, strain the water into a glass.

E. Drink the water on an empty stomach.

F. For extra help, you can grind the soaked seeds in a food processor.

G. Put this paste on your sore knee(s) for more pain relief.

Special Notes:

- Try warming the soaked water slightly before drinking for a comforting effect.
- Add a squeeze of lemon to the water to make it taste better and get an extra vitamin C boost.

28. Homemade Knee Soother - The Minty Clove Magic Rub

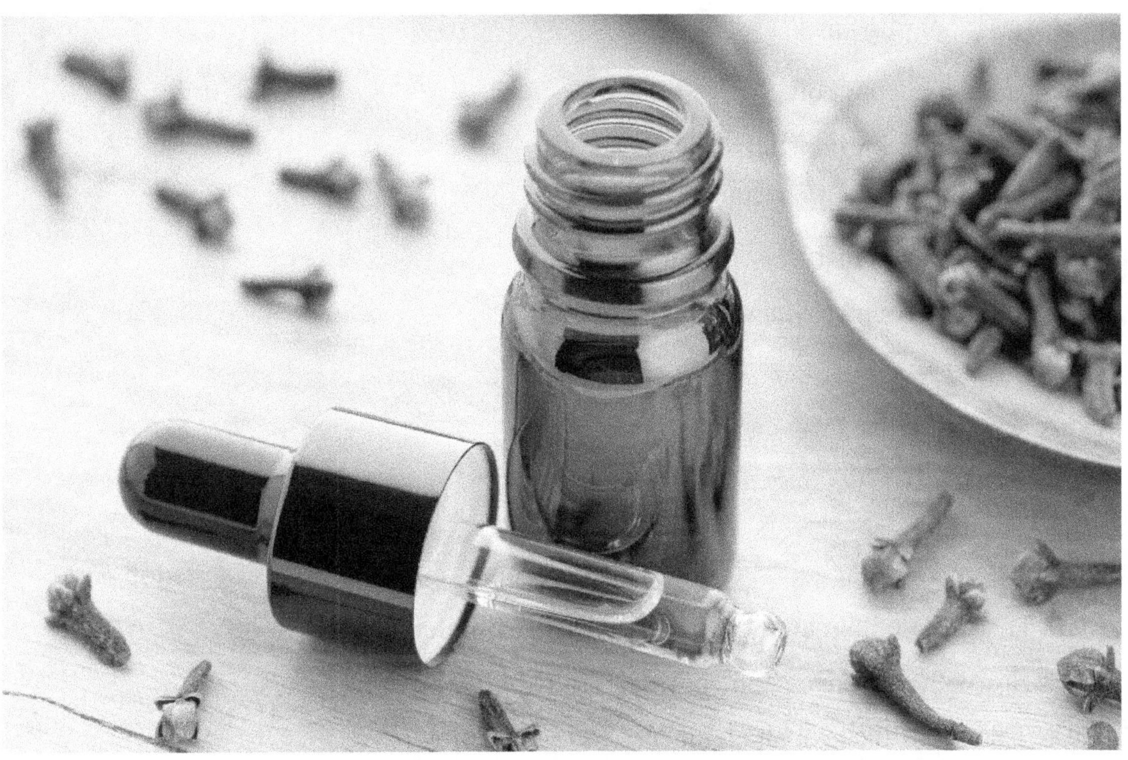

This DIY knee pain reliever is like a gentle Tiger Balm you can make at home. It's got a mix of oils that work together to ease aches. People love it because it's natural and smells nice. You can use it on your knees or other sore spots. It's pretty easy to whip up and works well for mild pain.

Preparation Time: 15 minutes

Serving size: 1 cup

Ingredients:

- 40 drops peppermint essential oil
- 40 drops eucalyptus essential oil
- 20 drops clove essential oil
- 3/4 cup olive oil
- 1/4 cup coconut oil
- 1/4 cup beeswax pellets
- 1 teaspoon vitamin E oil
- 10 drops rosemary essential oil
- 1 pinch ground cayenne pepper

xxxxxxxxxxxxxxxxxxxxxxxxx

Instructions:

A. Set up a double boiler. Mix olive oil, coconut oil, and beeswax in the top part.

B. Heat on medium until the beeswax melts completely.

C. Stir in the cayenne pepper.

D. Take it off the heat and let it cool for 5-8 minutes.

E. Add all the essential oils and vitamin E oil. Stir gently.

F. Pour the mix into a glass jar.

G. Let it sit until it turns solid.

H. To use, scoop a small amount with your fingers and rub it on your knee.

I. Close the jar tightly after each use. Keep it at room temperature.

Special Notes:

- For extra cooling, store the salve in the fridge. The cold feeling can help numb pain even more.
- If you want a smoother texture, strain out the cayenne pepper with a fine mesh sieve before adding the essential oils. This will give you all the heat without the grittiness.

29. Homemade Knee Soother: The Honey-Mustard Magic Cream

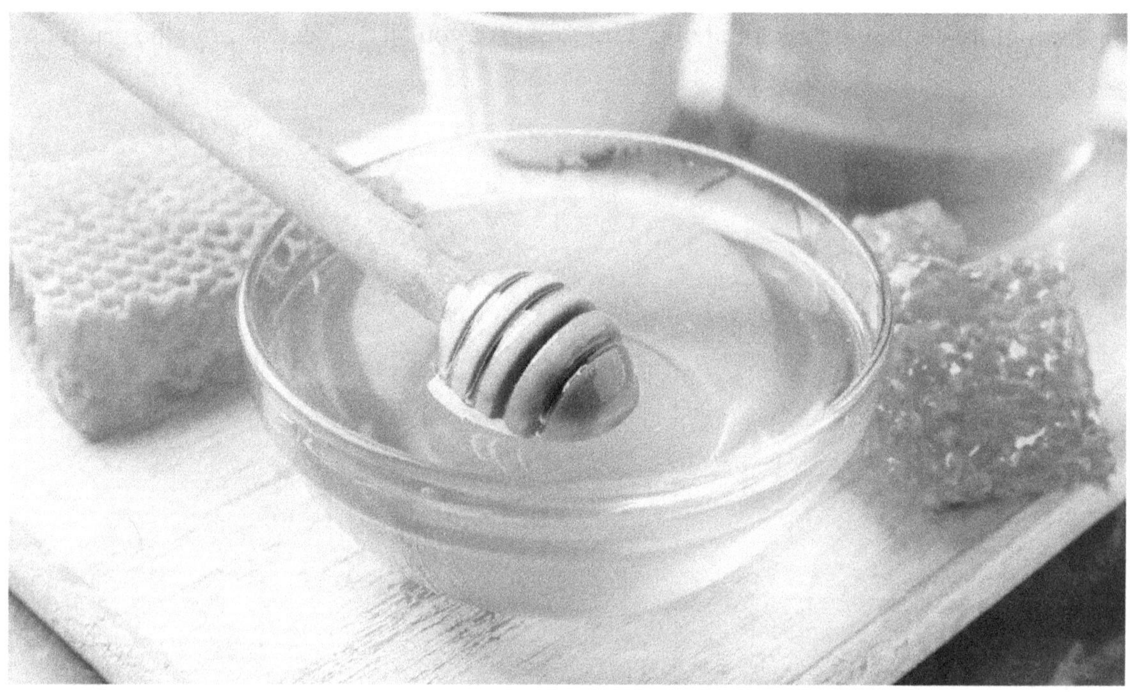

This simple home remedy helps ease knee and lower back pain. It's a mix of common kitchen items that work together to soothe aches from arthritis and joint issues. Easy to make and apply, it's a go-to for many looking for natural pain relief.

Preparation Time: 10 minutes

Serving size: 2 oz.

Ingredients:

- 1 tablespoon honey, pure
- 1 tablespoon mustard
- 1 tablespoon baking soda
- 1 tablespoon kosher salt

xxxxxxxxxxxxxxxxxxxxxxxx

Instructions:

A. Heat the mustard in a microwave-safe bowl.

B. Combine all ingredients in the bowl. Mix well until smooth.

C. If the baking soda fizzes when it meets the mustard, keep stirring. Mix for about 5-6 minutes.

D. Warm the cream slightly before use.

E. Spread the cream on your knee.

F. Cover with plastic wrap, then a clean towel.

G. Leave it on for at least 3 hours. You can also put it on before bed.

H. After treatment, take off the towel and wrap. Wash your knee with mild soap and warm water.

I. Use this remedy for 2-3 days to get the best results.

Special Notes:

- For extra soothing power, add a drop of peppermint oil to the mix. It gives a cool feeling that many find helpful for pain.
- If you're out of kosher salt, sea salt works too. Just make sure it's finely ground so it mixes well with the other ingredients.

30. Soothing Knee Rub - The Joint Whisperer

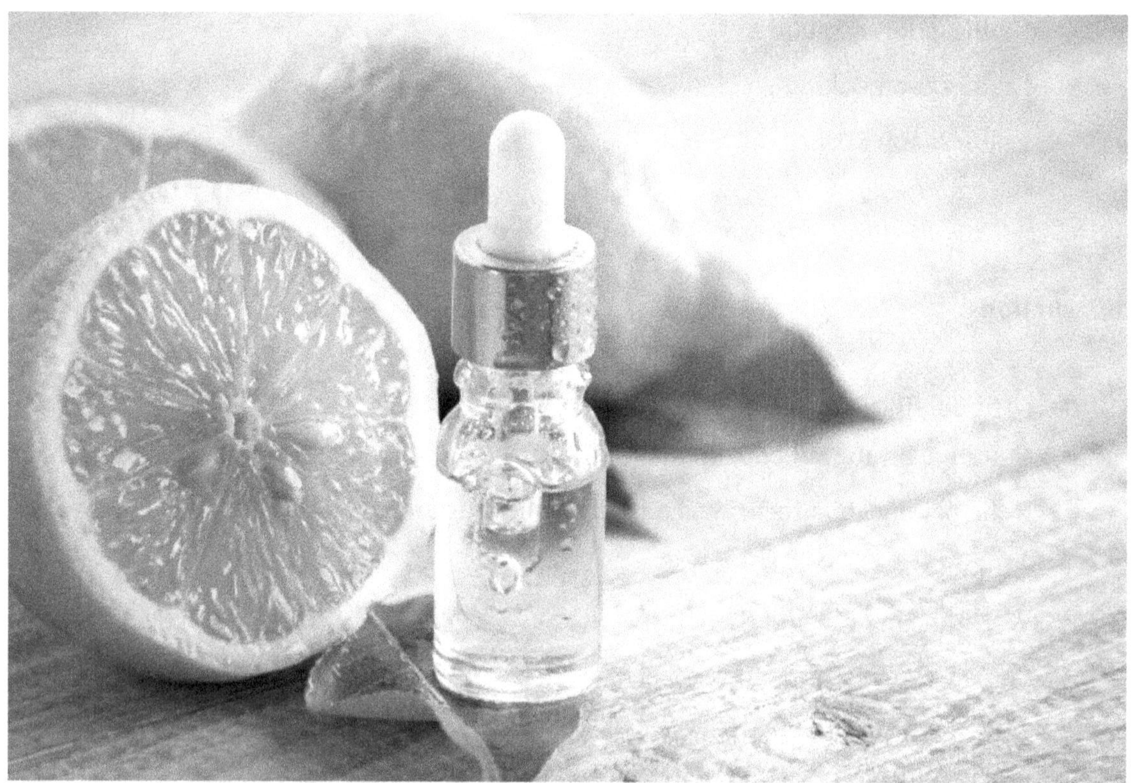

This homemade knee balm is a natural way to ease joint pain. It's popular among people who want to avoid harsh chemicals. Made with coconut oil and essential oils, it's easy to whip up at home. You'll love how it feels on your skin and how it helps with discomfort.

Preparation Time: 20 minutes

Serving size: 1/2 cup

Ingredients:

- 4 oz coconut oil
- 15 drops lavender essential oil
- 10 drops peppermint essential oil
- 10 drops eucalyptus essential oil
- 5 drops lemon essential oil
- 5 drops wild orange essential oil

xxxxxxxxxxxxxxxxxxxxxxxx

Instructions:

A. Put coconut oil in a mason jar.

B. Place the jar in a pan with warm water.

C. Heat on low until the oil melts.

D. Take the jar out of the water.

E. Add all the essential oils to the melted coconut oil.

F. Mix well.

G. Pour the mixture into small containers.

H. Let it cool to room temperature.

I. The balm will harden as it cools.

J. Apply to your knee area when needed.

K. Keep the container sealed if it's warm (75°F or higher) to prevent melting.

Special Notes:

- For an extra cooling effect, store the balm in the fridge. The cold temperature will give an added boost to the soothing properties.
- Try adding a few drops of ginger essential oil for its warming effect. It can help increase blood flow to the area and may provide additional pain relief.

31. Homemade Knee Soother (The Joint Whisperer)

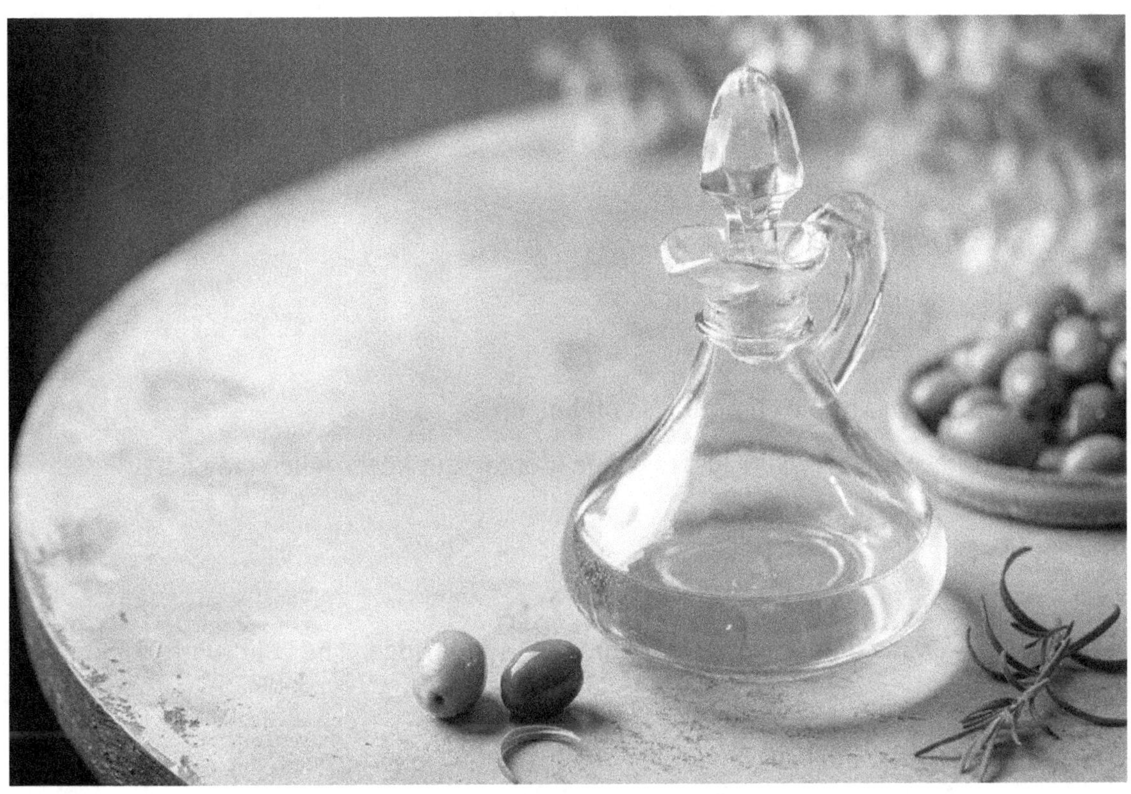

This simple rub is a lifesaver for achy knees. It's a go-to remedy, especially when your joints feel stiff from cold weather. Made with just two ingredients, it's quick to whip up and easy to use. People love how it warms and comforts sore spots without any fuss.

Preparation Time: 5 minutes

Serving size: 1/4 cup

Ingredients:

- 1/4 cup olive oil
- 1/2 teaspoon camphor essential oil

xxxxxxxxxxxxxxxxxxxxxxxxx

Instructions:

A. Get a small or medium glass container.

B. Pour the olive oil into the container.

C. Add the camphor essential oil.

D. Close the container tightly.

E. Shake the mixture well until it's combined.

F. Your knee rub is ready! Just massage it onto your knees when they hurt.

Special Notes:

- For an extra cooling effect, store the rub in the fridge. The cold rub feels amazing on hot, swollen knees.
- If you want a thicker consistency, melt 1 tablespoon of beeswax into the olive oil before adding the camphor. This makes it easier to carry in your bag without spills.

Conclusion

You've now explored a world of natural remedies for knee pain relief. These recipes offer a gentle, homemade approach to easing discomfort and improving joint health. From soothing balms to warming rubs, you have a variety of options to try.

Remember, these remedies aren't just for your knees. Many can be used for other aches and pains throughout your body. The skills you've learned here will serve you well beyond just knee care.

One of the best things about these recipes is how customizable they are. Feel free to adjust ingredients to suit your preferences or needs. You might find that a particular scent or herb works especially well for you.

Making your own pain relief products puts you in control of what goes on your skin. You can avoid harsh chemicals and know exactly what's in each remedy you use. This can be particularly comforting for those with sensitive skin or allergies.

Don't forget to share these recipes with friends and family who might benefit from natural pain relief. Spreading knowledge about homemade remedies can help many people find comfort without relying solely on over-the-counter medications.

As you continue to use these recipes, you may notice improvements in your overall joint health. Many of the ingredients used have benefits that go beyond just pain relief, supporting your body's natural healing processes.

Thank you for taking this journey into natural knee pain relief. We hope these recipes bring you comfort and ease in your daily life. Here's to healthier, happier knees and a more natural approach to pain management!

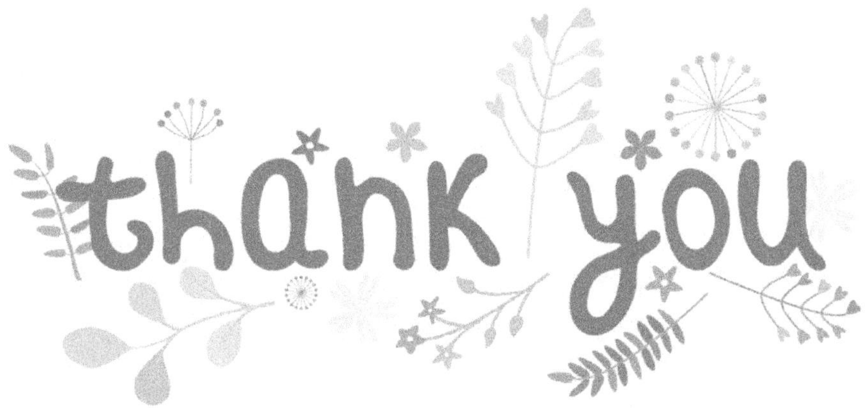

Dear Reader,

I want to express my sincere gratitude for downloading and dedicating your time to reading my book. It means the world to me that you chose to invest your valuable time in exploring the content I have shared. I truly hope that you found the information beneficial and that you had an enjoyable reading experience.

As an author, my primary goal is to impart my knowledge and insights to others. I recognize that there is an overwhelming number of e-books available, and I am deeply honored that you decided to give mine a chance. Your decision to read my work reflects your commitment to personal growth and learning, and I am thrilled to have played a role in your journey.

If you could spare a moment to provide an honest review or feedback about my book, I would be incredibly grateful. Your opinions and suggestions are invaluable to my development as a writer. They help me understand what resonates with readers and inspire me to create even more valuable content in the future. Who knows, your feedback might even spark the idea for my next book!

Once again, thank you for your support and dedication. It means more to me than words can express.

Martha Stanford